PRAISE FOR *CAGED LION*

"John Steel's vivid firsthand account of his unlikely friendship—and his life-changing workout routines—with the legendary Joseph Pilates reads like a ballet fairy tale. But it's all true. Steel recounts with verve (and admirable modesty) his own crucial role in assuring that the exercises Pilates used to heal famous dancers and ordinary New Yorkers alike would bloom into the worldwide wellness movement that millions know today."

> —Todd S. Purdum, author of *Something Wonderful: Rodgers and Hammerstein's Broadway Revolution*

"John Howard Steel from his unique perspective tells us about Joseph Pilates through the remembered lens of student, friend, and quasi family member of this brilliant, single-minded, destructively stubborn yet enigmatic creative force. John shares the barriers and legal hurdles that Pilates has overcome, many with John's unintentional leadership. John explains Pilates's enduring popularity from his fifty-seven years of being there. I highly recommend *Caged Lion*. It is an exciting, well-written, eye-opening story. As with a Pilates session, you will enjoy every minute of it and feel better for having read it."

> —Jim Henderson, former chairman and CEO of Cummins, Inc, and John's classmate at Culver and Princeton

"I binge-read in one sitting this engrossing biography of Joseph and Clara Pilates and the Pilates phenomenon written by a man who was not only a Pilates student for many years but also their friend. John Howard Steel is a great writer with a fascinating tale to tell!"

> —Anne Marie O'Connor, executive editor of *Pilates Style* magazine

"John has such a great writing voice. He doesn't waste words, is clear, funny, and able to efficiently paint vivid images with colorful vocabulary. I'm so happy how good this is and thankful it wasn't six hundred pages long. I believe it stands out from other Pilates books, because John is a wonderful storyteller. He knows how to tell a compelling story. Even his hypotheses and interpretations about Pilates are fascinating, humble, and insightful."

—Jeff Mizushima, writer, editor, producer

"A huge debt of gratitude is owed John Howard Steel, not only for his contribution to the Pilates method at a time when it wasn't clear if it would survive after Mr. Pilates death, but also for his delightful, insightful writing. Steel looks inside the complicated yet focused mind of Joseph Pilates and the behind-the-scenes life in his studio to provide the reader a deeper understanding of the man and his life's work. Thank you."

—Kevin A. Bowen, founder of The Pilates Method Alliance and
The Pilates Initiative; director, Core Dynamics Pilates, Santa Fe

"What an informative and fun read! Everybody will get something from this book: Pilates teachers and students and everyone who likes a good book. John Steel gives life to Joseph Pilates in ways that will only deepen your appreciation for or understanding of the method and the handful of people who saved it from sure extinction. This story is rich with suspense, intrigue, humor, and information about Joseph Pilates that you've never heard before. Some will find long-held notions completely upended in one sentence. Steel's writing style is clear, full of nuance and wit. I thoroughly enjoyed every page."

—Kristi Cooper, founder of Pilates Anytime

"*Caged Lion* is a fascinating story about the inside history of Pilates. John Howard Steel takes the reader on an extraordinary journey from first meeting Joseph Pilates in New York City to the global phenomenon that is modern-day Pilates. With a front-row seat, we're able to experience the ins and outs, ups and downs of moving Pilates from

a mom-and-pop enterprise into what it is today. As someone who started a fitness studio and someone who enjoys a good book, I loved this story of focus, passion, grit, and enterprise. Not to be missed."
—Elizabeth Cutler, cofounder and former CEO of SoulCycle

"*Caged Lion* is a story of two men: Joseph Pilates, who created a brilliant method of exercise, and the author John Howard Steel, who as Joseph's proxy, carried Joseph's vision and passion into what Pilates is today. Steel, from his unique perspective and deep personal connection, sets out a fascinating story of passion and perseverance. *Caged Lion* reads like a novel . . . a very, very good novel!"
—Shari Berkowitz, MS, *The Vertical Workshop's Pilates Teacher Blog*

C A G E D
L I O N

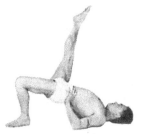

JOSEPH PILATES
& HIS LEGACY

J O H N   H O W A R D   S T E E L

Last Leaf Press

Published by Last Leaf Press, Santa Barbara, CA

Edited and designed by Girl Friday Productions
www.girlfridayproductions.com

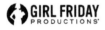

Photo editing: Lauren Steel
Cover design: Anna Curtis
Cover image: Courtesy of International Pilates University Fitness4you

ISBN (hardcover): 978-1-7334307-2-2
ISBN (paperback): 978-1-7334307-0-8
ISBN (ebook): 978-1-7334307-1-5

Library of Congress Control Number: 2020907493

CAGED
LION

CAGED LION

Nothing happens until something moves.

—Albert Einstein

CONTENTS

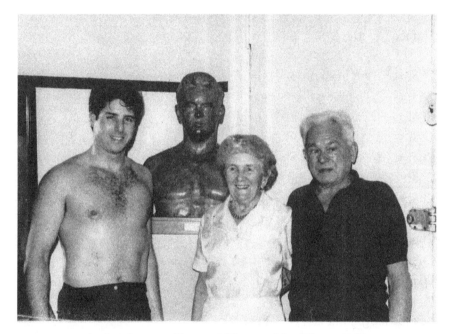

Author, bronze of Joe, and Clara and Joe Pilates, 1965.

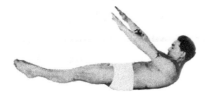

PREFACE

It was November 2007, and I was invited to be the keynote speaker before hundreds of teachers, studio owners, and other practitioners of Pilates at an early Pilates Method Alliance conference in Orlando, Florida. Joseph Pilates had been dead for forty years. During that time his exercise routine, which he had called "Contrology," had adopted the name "Pilates" and, after several rescues from near oblivion, was at last thriving. Over that long span of years I often thought of him, always with affection. I was still doing Pilates in a studio, with an instructor, once or twice each week. Hardly a session went by that my teacher didn't ask, "How would Joe Pilates have wanted you to do the exercise?" I loved the question. Sometimes, unasked, I volunteered: "This is the way Joe made everyone do it." My many and varied instructors, in France, England, New York, Colorado, and California, were a bit awed by, and quite proud of, teaching someone who had been originally taught by Joseph Pilates. And I remained moderately astounded that after the bizarre history of Pilates and the many years between then and now, and a vastly changed technological world, the movements of the exercise routine, the structure of the equipment, and the soul of Pilates were essentially as Joe had left them.

I had been out of the Pilates studio and business world, except as a client, since 1984, when the studio that I ran with Romana Kryzanowska in New York was sold to Aris Isotoner. I had become reinvolved in the 1990s when a new threat to Pilates arose—a claim of private ownership of the name Pilates by an entrepreneurial personal trainer supported by Romana. A hotly contested lawsuit ensued. That was resolved in 2000, and I again dropped below the radar and resumed the private role of student. I still loved taking lessons but had no interest in management.

I was honored, even touched, that the convention organizers had found me in Telluride, Colorado, and invited me to be their keynote speaker. The Pilates Method Alliance, or "PMA," was a new and wonderful organization that sought to standardize the teaching of Pilates and establish the requirements for teacher certification. It was a brave effort to get the rapidly expanding and uncontrolled world of Pilates under one roof, and to create a forum for the education, promotion, and requirements of Pilates training and instruction.

The keynote was on the evening of the first day. Many of the participants had spent a full day doing Pilates in various classes and were now relaxed and ready to learn a little about the history of their professional career choice. Some 450 people, all of whom were fit and vigorous, turned out in anticipation of the opening speech. My charge that evening was to sketch what it was like being taught Pilates by Joe Pilates, how the original studio had appeared and operated, and something about the man himself. I had a unique perspective. Only a few of us had lived long enough to know what it was like to be taught by the originator. Of these, I was the only amateur; the others were teaching professionals. These first-generation teachers were in the audience.

In the weeks before, as I prepared for my talk, my mind kept jumping to many questions: Who was this man I was to talk about? Where did he come from, and what inspired him to develop his exercise routine? I hadn't given a thought to these questions while Joe was alive. He never discussed his past or how he created his original exercise method of Contrology. In that aspect I was like everyone else: ignorant of the backstory behind both the man and his methods. When I began to outline my talk, my lack of knowledge of Joe's background scared me. I wondered how I could speak on a topic I knew little about. I certainly knew Joe as he was during the last little bit of his long and varied life. I knew what it was like doing Pilates under his watchful eye. And I knew him outside his gym. Yet, even with all the time I had spent with him, I knew no more of his past than anyone could find by punching his name into Google. And that was not much.

Recalling my time with Joe stimulated my curiosity. I wanted to know more about the central character in my talk. I wanted to know how Joe conceived of his exercise routine. I wondered what there was to the Pilates Method that suddenly caused it to burst forth from a small, almost cultlike following into a mass exercise program. And I had a further question—a personal question: What drove me over the years to keep Pilates afloat? How did I—someone who didn't make a career out of or even a dime from Pilates—get infected with the Joe bug? Sure, I wanted to have a place to do it, but when the corner pizzeria went out of business, I didn't learn how to run a pizzeria. Perhaps, doing this inquiry I might find out something about myself. There was a lot to cover and uncover here.

As I started my talk, I was curious how much my audience knew about the exercise regime they taught and had studied so intently. I asked: "Who in the audience knew that Pilates was the name of an actual person?" I was shocked when only half the audience raised their hands.

Next, I asked for a show of hands from those who knew that Pilates was a person and who thought he was alive. Half of those put their hands up. That left only 25 percent of the professionals in front of me who knew there was an individual named Pilates, and that he was no longer alive. I was taken aback. The man who'd given his name to a worldwide exercise phenomenon—people from forty-seven countries were attending this conference—was a virtual unknown to about 75 percent of the Pilates teachers in the audience.

I felt terrible. Joe had devoted his life to creating and teaching what was now a popular system of exercise to improve health and happiness, but the person named Pilates had been replaced by the exercise regime named Pilates. Joe had been lost to time, like an ancient city under the rubble of an advancing civilization.

I had trouble understanding how the Joe who had developed this program had slipped off the map. Maybe the history of the exercises was thought to be irrelevant to those learning to teach them. Probably no client ever asked about the source of what they were doing, so why waste precious class time on an unnecessary topic? When Joe was teaching me, I didn't ask where the idea for a movement or a piece of equipment came from. Following his instructions was hard enough. Maybe ignoring Joe lay with studio owners and teachers who were not exposed to the history or didn't care about it or didn't want to demystify their role as healers. Surprisingly, no one seemed to stop and consider that the man who conceived of this elaborate program might also have had very important insights into the exercises, how to teach them, and how to cue the student into performing them.

I quickly realized that my talk had a purpose. The people who had invited me sensed that their audience needed something more than a few laughs and quaint stories from an old man about another old man. Could be my audience would welcome insight into how the master taught Pilates. After all, they came to this convention to improve their teaching skills. Could be they also needed to understand what Joe thought was at the heart, the core, of his exercise program. Did Pilates have a soul? Was magic involved? If these were the questions my audience had, they were my questions as well.

I could feel the anticipation from the audience. They were all ears. I abandoned my outline and just started with the story of my relationship with Joe and his wife, Clara, and the Pilates exercises as Joe taught them. Oh well, I was accustomed to improvising. Every case I tried or appealed as a lawyer became an improvisation shortly after, if not during, the opening statement. Once I started to talk about Joe, I knew I was in a good place. I was at PMA to entertain and enlighten an audience about early Pilates as I remembered it. I hadn't been asked to talk about Joe's background or to give an inspirational chat—just to tell stories. Here I was, very emotional on realizing that right in front of me was the metamorphosis of an exercise routine Joe left in tatters forty years ago and living proof of its persistence through difficult times. Along with the proof of the success of Pilates evidenced by the large, eager crowd of professionals sitting in front of me came—in equal measure—how lost in all of this was Joe, the Thomas Edison of Pilates.

An hour passed in a flash. I stayed firmly on the side of the raconteur, telling funny stories about Joe and the shower, Joe and the gun, Joe at the zoo, Joe's gym-side manner, Joe walking on Eighth Avenue, and Joe smoking a cigar. Joe needed to be appreciated as a person, with all his skills and eccentricities. It was easy; it was fun; and when I looked out, I saw rapt attention. And there was welcome kindness when I tried to be funny. The talk just rolled along until the hotel's maintenance foreman interrupted me and said I had to end immediately because they needed to reconfigure the auditorium for the next event. The audience howled "No." The foreman called our event manager, who negotiated another forty-five minutes in the auditorium, much to the chagrin of the Teamster Union guys and the distress of my parched throat. The throat was lubricated with a glass of water. At the end of that next forty-five minutes, we had to leave. The audience was still hungry for stories and asked if I could go to the lobby and continue. I was flattered and pleased. They pulled over a chair for the old guy—me—while they, nimble and well-conditioned, sat on the floor. Another hour zipped by with questions and stories, my throat soothed this time by a beer or two. These people were starved for this stuff. And I was getting a kick out of telling Joe stories, many of which I hadn't thought about in decades.

The keynote address lasted almost three hours. I was very tired, in a good way, savoring how much pleasure I had from my trip down memory lane and how gratifying it was to see the enthusiastic reaction. I had started with this sad feeling that poor Joe had been discarded, thrown on the ash heap, and I ended with the sense that if he were brought back into historical focus, he would be well received.

People needed to know about him. They wanted to connect the dots of the Pilates tradition back to the beginning. And I hadn't even touched the first eighty years of his life.

Over the next three days of the convention, during which I had nothing official to do, I was constantly surrounded by teachers from all over the country, and some from as far away as Russia and Japan, who had questions about Joe or just wanted to sit around and listen to more stories. I had a lovely entourage everywhere I went, and I thoroughly enjoyed the attention. I spent time with several first-generation teachers, who were very curious about the Joe outside the gym even though they had studied with him. They also enjoyed hearing a perspective on his teaching from someone not in training to teach.

From the reaction to my talk, and the reaction to many similar talks at subsequent conferences, it was obvious there was a thirst for information about Joe, about the genesis of Pilates, what Joe and Pilates were like back then, and how it survived Joe's death and became so popular; people were even hungry for gossip. They wanted to hear it all from one of the few surviving students taught by Joe, who also became a social friend, Clara's lawyer, and a pivotal person in the forty years between Joe's death and this convention. Many attendees said the same thing: "You should write a book."

So I did. Here it is, thirteen years later. Much of what occurred over the many years of this story I vividly recalled. Remembering certain details was challenging. And as I drilled deeper into Joe's own story, starting with the popular version, I discovered huge gaps about his early years. He was not one to talk about his past. He left no diary, journal, correspondence, or any other trace. A German immigrant, he passed through his early life, before he reached the United States, without leaving footprints. No one had Joe's story. Everyone thought they did, but even under the dimmest of lights, the popular version didn't hold together.

The real story of Joe's early years, if it was to be part of a book—and I certainly thought that to be essential—had to come from me. As a student and friend of Joe's, I had a special vantage point. Digging and thinking were my stock in trade as a litigator, and I hope they served me well in filling gaps by bridging the holes with solid information.

I researched, thought about, and approached Joe's background as if it were a crime scene. There were clues that could be pieced into a coherent and plausible story, but I can't swear to the accuracy or the validity of some of my insights and conclusions.

Despite the impossibility of verifying everything, I think it fair to call this a true story. The people, the dates, the places, and my own activities are recounted here to the best of my recollection. Many of the explanations and reconstructions of historical events were pieced together from known facts, circumstances, and probabilities. For Joe's early history, I depended on the research of others, who are given credit in the narrative. Where I lacked an explanation of Joe's actions or an insight into his motives, I tried to see them as Joe might have seen them, based on my general familiarity with his outlook on life.

Some of my conclusions will challenge long held and widely accepted beliefs. I hope I have sufficiently explained how I arrived at these conclusions to at least get you, the reader, thinking. Some of the portrayals of principal actors may upset readers who know these individuals in a context different from mine. Professionals and even students may disagree with the reasons I have given for the enduring popularity of Pilates. I understand and accept all of that and say, in my defense, I tried hard to connect the dots, which I acknowledge required a stretch here and there.

John Howard Steel, Santa Barbara, March 2020

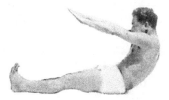

CHAPTER 1

An Inauspicious but Important Beginning

Early one brisk fall morning in 1963, I left my apartment on upper Fifth Avenue, New York City, took the bus downtown to 57th Street, and walked west across town until I reached a shabby, old-style New York tenement, fronting on an entire block. I was on my way to a physical therapist highly recommended by my mother. Mom had been hounding me for at least six months to see him. She thought this man was a wizard with the human body and was certain that he could fix my chronic stiff neck. I was skeptical—just another of my mother's many enthusiasms. My resistance finally cracked not so much to relieve the pressure on my neck as to end the pressure from my mother.

I entered the unlocked outer door of 939 Eighth Avenue and stepped into a cramped, smelly space serving as the lobby, mail room, laundry drop-off, umbrella shake-out room, and entry hall for the occupants of the many small apartments. The inner-door latch was broken and provided as much security as a sign saying: "Thieves Not Admitted."

Even though unnecessary, I hit the buzz-me-in button next to a faded "Pilates" label. Might as well let this Mr. Pilates know I was on time. Then I walked up the main stair to the second floor and through the heavy fire door into a dim hall where, to my surprise, a barely clothed old man stood like a statue. He had to be Joseph Pilates, the miracle-working physical therapist. He was deeply tanned and had an impressive head of unkempt white hair. To the extent he had on clothes, they were his work outfit: tight black shorts and canvas slippers. He was topless despite—or in defiance of—the chilly November cold in the hall. Long, loosely hanging but very muscled arms showed veins popping out everywhere. He wore thick glasses in nondescript plastic frames with tape on one temple. Behind the lenses, his left eye was fixed on me while his right eye was immobile. It was glass. He was several inches shorter than me and very compact. His stance—balanced, upper body forward, arms up—was that of a boxer ready for a fight. The picture that popped into my mind was of a lion with a great mane, on its hind legs, paws up. Vigor and energy poured out of him. The man I was facing radiated the authority of a Marine drill sergeant, and some of the meanness too.

"Mr. Pilates?" I asked, just to be sure. "Hello."

I took his extended hand, which he stuck out into the considerable space between us without so much as a smile. The handshake was weird. He seemed to be checking my pulse. He not only had a finger on my inner wrist, his left eye scanned me up, down, and sideways as if I were an applicant for a job where appearance and personal hygiene were important. He held the handshake an uncomfortably long time.

I was a product and member in good standing of the very comfortable American middle class. Yet here I stood in a seedy hallway, face-to-face with a mostly naked man who was fifty-two years my senior and from another world, and I, the highly educated and socially adept New York lawyer, was off balance—not a good thing when facing someone with the stance and demeanor of a boxer. I tried to break through the icy welcome of Mr. Pilates by explaining why I was there. He grunted an unmistakable signal that warned me: Mr. Pilates was not interested in talk of any kind.

At the very least, I expected questions about my health and what I thought I needed from him—the sorts of questions that physical therapists should ask. I thought he might mention my mother and father, who were his clients. Nothing, just a tense silence. His face reflected neither warmth nor hostility. Only intensity. My discomfort grew. My Ivy League schooling, properly fitting suit, spiffy shirt and tie, and shined shoes didn't matter at all here. I felt very much out of place. But I didn't leave.

I followed Joe through an old-fashioned door with a large opaque glass panel on which was painted in beautiful script "Joseph H. Pilates." This was the gym. It was approximately fifteen feet wide and twenty long—the size of an old New York apartment living room, which it had been at one time—with a high ceiling and three tall windows facing east on Eighth Avenue. Even with all the morning light streaming in, the room had a dark, heavy, Teutonic look. Worn Oriental rugs covered most of the floor. The walls, café au lait colored from paint or age, were covered from floor to ceiling with pictures of Joe doing the exercises. All the photographs had an antique appearance in dark frames hung precisely edge to edge.

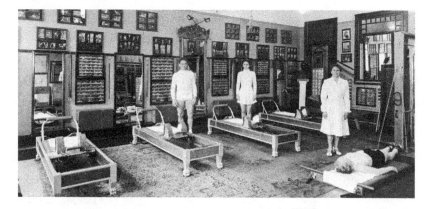

Joe's gym around 1940. From left: Joe Pilates, his niece Mary Pilates, Clara Pilates, and an unknown client.

The atmosphere of the gym was comforting. There was something warm and welcoming about the space: the openness and the décor. What caught my eye was what I guessed to be the exercise equipment: apparatus unlike anything I had ever seen before was lined up with military precision like jeeps in an army motor pool, taking up most of the huge floor. Four central pieces resembled single beds, with sturdy frames of nicely burnished wood and carved claws where the legs met the floor. These well-made and polished pieces almost looked comfortable until I examined them closely. Each frame supported a platform—like a bed frame supporting a mattress—that was upholstered in black leather. The platform was about four feet long and went back and forth inside the frame on wheels at each corner. Four long springs connected the platform to one short side of the frame. Belting-leather straps, looped through pulleys, were attached to the platform in opposition at the other end. Pull on the straps at one end and the springs at the other exerted an equal and opposite force. The leather straps and other pieces of industrial-strength hardware looked like restraints or torture devices.

As I soon learned, these contraptions, the centerpiece array in the gym, were called "Universal Reformers," the Pilates signature machine known the world over now as "the Reformer." Another contraption in the shape of a wooden chair sat in the corner. It was unremarkably named "the Chair," and it had a discomforting resemblance to an electric chair. Yet another piece, called a "Ladder Barrel," left nothing to conjecture: its design almost spoke to you—your body would be draped over it. I could hear my spine snapping. One device named "the Spine Corrector" took up little space. I suspected it was there to put your back together after the Ladder Barrel. Another bit of gear had the oh-so-friendly moniker "the Guillotine." Nowhere in this array could I see any of the equipment you might expect in a gym in 1963—no weights, barbells, medicine balls, or chin-up bars. Joe sensed my bewilderment and said: "I invented all this equipment to teach Contrology. That is all we do here. That is all you need for your life. You will see."

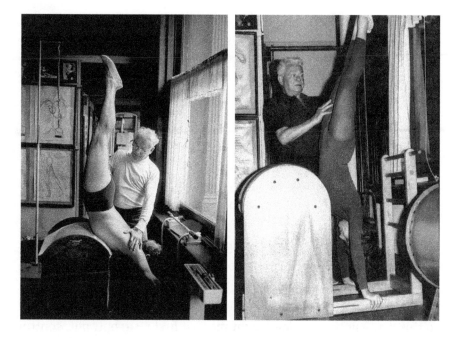

Joe spots the author's parents, Arthur and Ruth Steel, over the Ladder Barrel.

Despite the off-putting apparatus, the room appeared neat and precisely organized; it smelled of furniture polish, leather, floor wax, and a healthy dose of three-in-one oil. Here and there among the photos of Joe demonstrating the exercises, like early stop-action pictures, were large headshots and full-body photos of him in various poses, all in black-and-white faded to a sepia tone. In a corner stood a bronze statue of Joe, about two feet tall, on a pedestal in the pose of an ancient Greek discus thrower. Like classical Greek athletes, the statue was unclothed and anatomically correct. There was a full-size bronze head of Joe against a wall. No question this was Joe's gym.

Joe handed me a pair of skimpy canvas ballet slippers, without asking me about size, and ordered: "You wear these, no socks." Then he asked: "Did you bring trunks and a towel?"

"Yes."

"Go in there, change, and come out." He pointed to a plastic shower curtain. Two or three words fell from my mouth as I started to tell Mr. Pilates about my stiff neck. He looked at me as if I hadn't heard his instructions and repeated "Go change." I went behind the shower curtain into a room little bigger than a walk-in closet. A pre-fab shower, like ones found in every cheap motel, filled half the space. This was the "men's locker room," a primitive, makeshift space lacking lockers and room. Better it should have been called the "men's changing closet."

When I returned to Joe, wearing only my skimpy shorts—like today's running shorts—I felt exposed even though my body was trim and athletic. Joe pointed to a Universal Reformer. A name of ominous portent: reform like in reform school, the worry of every child?

Joe told me to sit down at a specific spot on the Reformer, and then before I started to lower myself, he gave me terse but clear instructions: "Push your backside out, arms go forward, eyes up, resist gravity." I had to sit two or three times before doing it to his satisfaction. What was this? Had I come here to get corrected on my sitting technique? Yet to this day, I sit the way Joe taught me that first visit: butt out, control through the stomach all the way down.

Once I sat to Joe's satisfaction (a prerequisite to proceeding to the next step), he gave me a long instruction. "You now have to lie on the Reformer, and you have to do it the right way, same every time. Here's how: pull up the knees to your chest with your stomach muscles, lean back while you twist to the right, straighten the legs, put your feet on the bar, your head between the shoulder rests, relax your spine, and breathe."

Going from sitting to lying down should be a snap, right? Something we all do every day getting into bed. Just coordinate a ninety-degree turning movement with lifting my legs and then lower my body simultaneously. The precise spot where I sat on the Reformer had to be located so my head would fall on the headrest and between the shoulder restraints. But what seemed like it would be easy wasn't. Each attempt was followed by: "Okay, good, now try again, smoothly." All this just to lie down.

I kept at it until I didn't get a "try again," and we proceeded to the next little movement. I thought this was nonsense—a waste of my time. I wasn't getting any exercise, much less doing anything that could help my stiff neck. Consciously engaging my stomach to raise my legs was a new one. Never did that before; I just raised them.

Despite my skepticism, I followed Joe's instructions to the letter. The movements were all basic. And I was relieved because his directions were short and clear. Executing them smoothly, however, wasn't easy. Joe had my full attention like a dog to its master. I was tuned to his voice, waiting for his next directive. But once we got past the "getting in position correctly" phase—no more than five minutes—and started actual exercises on this contraption, everything changed. The movements ceased being familiar. The exercises required pushing against a specific number of springs (which I had to attach) or pulling on straps (which I had to get my feet into or grip) in all kinds of strange, but never uncomfortable, positions. It was like driving a rental car for the first time in Great Britain and being faced with a clockwise traffic circle. Nothing clicked in. My brain was jammed, and all my neural channels were occupied simply following orders. Joe's instructions were bare bones but enough. He said, "Do this" or "Do that," and I did it immediately without thinking or questioning why.

Even with all the repetition to get it right, we moved through the routine at a snappy pace, with no pauses. Joe was like a metronome for exercise: hypnotic. I got in a groove. To do what he asked, I had to tense some muscles, relax other muscles, breathe at the right time, and keep my mind focused on the movement of the moment and suppress all unrelated thoughts. This was far different from the rest of my day, where my brain seemed crammed with stuff demanding my attention. Whatever I might have expected as "exercise," this wasn't it. I didn't even notice my neck. I was in a state of suspended consciousness.

Joe took me through a series of separate exercises stitched together as one continuous routine. Changing my position on the apparatus for the next exercise was part of the routine. Setting up the springs, straps, and carriage bed for the next exercise, which everyone did for themselves, was also part of the routine. There was a lot to keep in mind and no space to think about anything else.

Each exercise had a name. Some were descriptive, many whimsi-cal. The exercises I did on that first day and continue to do to this day had names such as "the Hundred," "Rocker with Open Legs," "Rolling Like a Ball," "Horse," "Frog," "Crab," "Spine Stretch," "the Saw," and "the Corkscrew." Joe announced each name as he told me what to do. The name connected me to the exercise, the setup, and its order. He never once demonstrated how to do anything. He was the opposite of the maxim, "show, don't tell." There were approximately fifty exer-cises, organized in sets of four or five movements requiring little or no change of position or adjustments to the apparatus within that set. The sets, like the individual exercises, had a descriptive name. For example, the beginning set was "Leg Work." Another set would be "Long Box," then "Short Box." The set and exercise names were an excellent asso-ciative device, and to this day the same names are used by all Pilates teachers.

As if these strange movements weren't enough for the first day, all the while I was moving my body to his commands, Joe was telling me when to breathe. And that he did in his inimitable German-accented English: "Breeze the air in; breeze the air out."

Normally, when doing strenuous exercise, even aerobics, the deci-sion about when to inhale and exhale is made unconsciously by our very sensitive and complex oxygen-regulating system. This system, which measures the oxygen in blood and seeks to increase or decrease it depending on input from other organs (and you thought your smart-phone was genius!), works in the background to cause us to breathe faster and deeper when our bodies need oxygen. You feel it working, like you used to feel the automatic shift in the car going through the gears. But unlike the driver of a car, your body can't anticipate future demand. But your brain can, and Joe could. So Joe wanted me to take control of this vital but usually ignored function of breathing not only to take care of my body's need for oxygen, but to prepare it for what was coming. Just like a race-car driver shifting up for a straightaway and down going into a turn.

Joe knew breathing could be better regulated with the conscious mind in control, based principally on what the body was doing. He

forced me to visualize my lungs like a bellows. Did the movement of
the exercise expand the rib cage? Was the abdomen making room
for the diaphragm? Hard to inhale when compressing the lungs. Joe's
override of my reflexive breathing worked. His timing was better than
my body's automatic control. I was neither breathless nor straining to
hold my breath. The breathing was tuned to the movement. Breathing
now became one more thing to think about. While the timing of my
breathing was under my control, the depth was determined automatically by my need for oxygen. Timing my breathing by attaching it
to movement was much easier than I would have expected. Joe had
me breathing semiconsciously by using my body motion to assist the
inhales and exhales: any movement contracting the chest forced an
exhale, while movement expanding the chest assisted the inhale. I was
moving more air in and out of my lungs with ease.

At the time, I was a very preppy young lawyer trained during my
entire life to perform to the best of my ability whatever was asked of
me, whether in school, in sports, in the army, at work, or socially. And
I had developed what I thought were tried-and-true techniques to
do okay in each situation. I paid close attention. I memorized. I took
notes. I studied the notes. I practiced. I tried to understand. My techniques had served me well. I got good grades, played on varsity teams,
survived combat engineer basic training, and had a good job. And here
I was in a very strange room with an odd man giving me a boatload of
choreography for an exercise program like nothing I had ever experienced. All to be done thoughtfully and properly in a coordinated and
smooth manner on "machines" requiring complicated and continuous
adjustments.

There was one more disorienting requirement. I was forbidden to
take notes, to memorize, even to repeat the names of the exercises.
When Joe caught me trying to "learn," which he did frequently just by
observing my furrowed brow, he got very irritated and told me not to
try to remember anything. He said my body would do it automatically.
He wouldn't repeat the name of the exercise if I asked him. All my
so-called good study habits were now out the window, forbidden—at
least for this endeavor.

How was I going to impress Joe and show him what a smart learner I was without my usual crutches? I was cornered. I had to trust him. I had to give up thinking about what I was doing and just do it. That was enough. I realized I was being trained like a circus animal, not taught like a student, although without treats (or even a pat on the back) when I did something correctly. But was I learning? Didn't matter; there was no test, and that alone was a relief. There was no need to anticipate, no need to memorize with the hope it stuck.

Suddenly, with no warning, Joe said, "Okay, finished, shower and change."

By this time, I was running on fumes yet had no idea when the session would be over. I was thrilled, like when the drilling stops at the dentist. Normally, when uncomfortable experiences are over, one relaxes, drops the shoulders, takes a deep breath, unclenches the hands, and wiggles the toes to shake off the tension. No need to do this after a session with Joe. To my surprise, I was already relaxed.

The session lasted about forty-five minutes. I had kept going throughout. I never felt physically unable to do what Joe instructed although it was tough keeping up toward the end. Time had passed quickly because I wasn't thinking about what I was doing as exercise. Rather, I wasn't thinking at all—just doing.

When it was over, I was suddenly tired way down deep, soaked with sweat, somewhat dazed, and critically nauseous. I raced for the changing room and no sooner did I get there than I threw up in the shower stall (there was no toilet or sink). An okay location (the only one) to vomit: plenty of water and a drain. I got it all cleaned up using my sweaty towel. I showered and tried to cool down. I was moving slowly. Joe's routine had sucked my energy stores dry.

I was showered, but still dripping wet—the little towel was unusable. And still sweating. I was hungry and thirsty, too, with vomit breath, dressed for work feeling I should undress to take another shower. I made a mental note to bring two big, clean towels next time—if there was to be a next time. I got back into my business clothes, which once on were no wetter than after a packed ride on the New York subway during a heat wave before air-conditioning. In other words, soaking wet.

As I walked past Joe on the way out, he said: "Shoulders back and down, chin up, head back. See you day after tomorrow, seven o'clock. Five dollars."

Joe spoke as if I were a longtime regular who had committed to this program. I nodded a yes, trying not to exhale so he wouldn't smell the vomit on my breath. I had a toothbrush in my office, but until then, I stunk. As I left the gym, still dazed, my body felt like it had been put through an old-fashioned, hand-cranked laundry wringer like in the Bugs Bunny cartoons. I felt taller. Even my neck was relaxed. I suspected the stiff neck might be gone forever even though I could recall no exercise dealing with my neck. I took the elevator down, not trusting my legs.

When I got outside and regained a tolerable amount of composure, I reviewed this unexpected experience. I was surprised that Joe Pilates had any clients. How did my mother and father get through this routine? My massive disorientation, nausea, and deep fatigue sent me quite a message. Something astonishing had occurred. What it was on one level—my physical condition—was obvious. I was not nearly as fit as I thought. What the experience was on another level—how I felt about it—was murky. When I had arrived at the gym just an hour earlier, I was a cocky amateur athlete who thought he was in great shape, except for the chronic stiff neck. When I left an hour later, I was limp as a dishrag with bad breath and a smelly towel in my gym bag. But my body seemed happy even if I was out of sorts. Barely noticeable was a release of tension around my shoulders and neck.

Not only was I physically drained, I was emotionally shaken. An hour or so earlier right before I met Joe, I was determined to reject him as a quack. I didn't need a trainer or want to go to a gym. Now after a bizarre workout I had agreed, without a thought, to return for more at seven o'clock in the morning two days hence. If others had an initiation even close to mine, there had to be something about him that attracted and kept clients.

I wondered whether Joe had been testing me. Looking back, I suspect he was. At this point in his life, Joe no longer devoted time to anyone not committed to his work. To weed out those he didn't want to bother with, he drove hard from the start with everyone. Maybe he super challenged those he prejudged as dilettantes. I had to be in the "perceived as a dilettante" category. I can imagine what Joe saw when he first looked at me. If he detected my attitude, and I suspect he did, he had to pick up on my arrogance and sense of superiority. I dressed as a young, successful lawyer. The suit fit perfectly, shirt had that custom-made tailoring, French cuffs with gold cuff links, shoes very English and highly polished, and the carefully selected and knotted tie pulled it all together. Joe could tell immediately that I came from a world removed from his.

Many months later, on one of my arm-in-arm walks with Joe down Eighth Avenue, he told me it was good I vomited that first time. I was surprised and embarrassed that he knew. Joe said the physical exertion did not cause it. "Not to vurry; it vas good," he told me. "You have more than vomit to get out of your body."

What did Joe Pilates know that I didn't? Who was he?

***

I was dazed after my first session with Joe Pilates; I felt like I had survived a near car crash. But now I was safe, back on familiar New York streets. I was headed to work—a place where I felt secure, a place I felt in control and a place where I knew what I had to do and was confident I could do it. I didn't want to think about the experience with Joe, so I tried to push it from my mind.

Except I couldn't. I had been drawn to Mr. Pilates, his weird gym and routine, for reasons I didn't then understand. Was I attracted to torture? Maybe I simply made a mistake? But it didn't feel like any of that. It felt like I wanted to go back. There was something there, up in that gym with that old man, that I needed. And if I had to sweat to get it: a small price to pay. It wasn't just the exercise, or the stretching, or the endorphin rush. It was something about Joe and something he buried in the routine. This attraction was irrational; nothing added up. Listening to the pull in my gut was not how I had decided to do most everything in my life. I was a balance-the-pros-and-cons kind of guy, and usually the strongest pro, the one that got two votes, was that it was *expected* of me. This was different; I couldn't even discern any pro. I just sensed I would be back in Joe's gym for another session. Of course I had no idea that the future of Pilates hung on my decision.

Despite knowing deep down I would return, I spent the next two days questioning my unhesitating nod of the head when Joe invited me back. Had Joe taken control of me in forty-five minutes? Had I become Joe's Manchurian Candidate so quickly? Or was I just so tired or disoriented that I lost my senses?

I could always cancel. It wasn't as if I were going to the electric chair. I didn't even know Joe's phone number and would have to get it from my mother—and explain. A hurdle. But did I need to put myself through yet another torturous experience? Wasn't living in New York, marriage, and practicing law enough? I knew I was missing something: Is that why I had impulsively nodded okay? There was this strange pull. I was experiencing a weird sensation: I was sinking in deep water, or quicksand, and needed air, and I just had to stay up long enough to grab a lifesaving ring thrown to me.

I had to stop the back-and-forth in my head and get on with my life. And there was something an experienced lawyer had impressed upon me about always keeping my options open even if I am certain I don't need to. If I didn't go back, my experience with Pilates would be finished. If I did go back, my option to continue or quit remained open. And maybe I could find out something about myself . . . why I was attracted to this craziness like the moth to the flame.

Two mornings later I got out of bed far too early and headed out the door. Like all early rising New Yorkers hanging on a strap in a hot, crowded bus, I was in a detached mental state, neither enthusiastic nor resistant. But unlike most of my fellow passengers, I wasn't going to work. I was going to a gym looking and feeling like a pack mule, with an overflowing briefcase hanging off one shoulder and my gym bag in the other hand stuffed with clean shorts, my new ballet workout slippers, and two large towels. Hanging from the strap alerted me to some residual soreness in my shoulder and chest, undoubtedly from Session 1. The soreness felt good, like I had used a muscle or two.

In the bus I tried to remember what I could about Session 1, in preparation for Session 2. I wanted to look good, and preparation was the key to that. But I couldn't remember the details of any exercise. Now and then a name like "the Hundred," "the Teaser," or "Rolling Like a Ball" stuck in my mind. I recalled Joe's insistence on the one way to do not only the exercises but things like sitting and changing positions. I was ready once again to pay close attention to the instructions. And who could forget the messy ending? I pictured Joe standing over me, telling me what to do. I couldn't remember what he told me; that was a blur.

When I arrived at 939, I went right into the vestibule without pushing the buzzer. The building entrance was just as grubby as it had been two days earlier, but my eyes overlooked what on day one had been startling. This time I took the decrepit elevator. I was only going up one floor—a short fall if the cable broke. Lo and behold: the elevator ascended smoothly and stopped dead level with the second floor.

In the gym, the lights were on. A deep quiet hung over the place. Joe, alone, was bent over and fiddling with a machine, dressed in black trunks and canvas slippers, this time with a white turtleneck. The emptiness was eerie, like arriving at a theater two hours before showtime and catching someone onstage, sweeping. Joe looked like a gnome with his compact body, long arms, and slightly bowed but very muscular legs. He seemed less aggressive than at our first encounter although not friendly. After all, he was about to torture me.

When I said, "Good morning, Mr. Pilates," he barely looked up. It was as if I had disrupted the silence that permeated the room. His brief glance, as I learned, was Joe's customary response to "Hello," if you could call it a response. This less-than-welcoming greeting never changed over the years I knew him. Joe's affect conveyed: "You are here to work, so get with it."

If Joe was surprised or glad to see me, he didn't reveal it. The impersonal greeting was a slap to my ego. I had worked so hard at my first session, I wanted, and expected, a pat on the back. I thought he would appreciate that I did him the honor of coming back. But Joe was not about to say anything to massage my delicate ego. His presence and readiness to teach me his program—his prescription for taking care of myself—were the extent of his demonstration of appreciation for my return.

I had before me an eighty-year-old man about to focus on me and exert a lot of energy and time to teach me a system he believed would improve the rest of my life. He had invited me back after the introductory session. What more did I want? Even though Joe was not into grades, I seemed to have passed an unknown test, or was that just me thinking everything was a test? Maybe it was not a test. Maybe Joe just wanted another client? But I didn't yet know Joe. It took me quite a while to learn that true appreciation was not just a few common words easily spoken. It took even longer to accept that doing my best was enough.

Shortly after I entered the gym, an old, very thin woman with glasses slipped in silently and ghostlike. In contrast to Joe, she was pure white from head to toe: white nurse's dress buttoned up the front that came down to her ankles, white stockings, practical white leather shoes, white hair, white skin. Very antiseptic, like the movie stereotype of a trilingual nurse at a tuberculosis sanatorium high in the Alps.

Joe introduced the lady in white as Clara, his wife and assistant. He told Clara I was the son of Ruth and Arthur, without mentioning my name, but remembering theirs. Clara quietly said, "Hello," extending her bony hand and giving me a faint smile. I could barely see her eyes behind her thick glasses. I recall her face being friendly. Joe indicated the pleasantries were over; time to get back to work.

Through the plastic curtain and into the men's locker room I went. Off with my business clothes, on with the shorts and canvas shoes, and back out, towel in hand, ready to face the master. I was nervous like I used to get in high school, preparing to wrestle a very buff, long-limbed steel worker's son from Gary, Indiana, with cauliflower ears and a state champ patch on his warm-up jacket. My wrestling coach said that pre-match nervousness was good: adrenaline and all that. Maybe this Pilates nervousness was also "good," even though it was uncomfortable.

I stepped out of the locker room wearing my confident face. I couldn't let Joe see me so messed up. Underneath this false front, I was desperately trying to remember what to do, where to start. Joe pointed to a Universal Reformer and I dropped my butt onto the apparatus at the spot where I remembered starting last time. I swung my legs around and put my feet up on the bar to get into the supine position. My head ended up in the right spot on the machine. How lucky!

Getting properly positioned was a good start. My body had remembered something. I was impressed with myself; Joe was unmoved. Other instructions from Session 1 occasionally popped up as Session 2 proceeded. Joe was the same as before; I was a lot more relaxed. After all, I was now there voluntarily. Even though he didn't dispense compliments, he didn't criticize or negatively correct me. His instructions were always positive: "Do this" instead of "Don't do that!" So different from most athletic coaches who focused on what you did wrong. What a relief.

While I was doing one exercise, I couldn't remember what came next, so I gave up trying and stuck to concentrating on what I was doing. Bits and pieces of each exercise felt familiar: just enough to let me know I could learn it without actively memorizing. Finally I turned off my inner student. It was so much easier not to think. Joe was there to tell me how to adjust the springs, what straps to use, and what movements the exercise required. He made no move to help even when I was having difficulty following his instructions. He didn't adjust the apparatus or help me get into position. He watched calmly as I struggled with very unfamiliar adjustments, but he kept me moving in a rhythm he chose, like an orchestra conductor. There were no starts, no stops, no breathers: continuous movement at a steady pace, like a jog between a walk and a run.

I fell into his rhythm. And his control of my breathing felt right. He never explained why I had to inhale or exhale at a certain time, but my body seemed to agree with him. Now and then I got into a breathing groove, inhaling and exhaling in sync with the exercise. When that happened, Joe stopped telling me when to breathe. I never strained to grab air or felt short of breath. Because of the pace and the breathing,

I was able to relax and work hard without straining, which was good, considering the sweat pouring out of me.

Finally Joe said, "Finished." I showered and dressed. At least this time I didn't throw up. As on day one, much of what I did in that session didn't stick in my mind. I left the locker room with a bounce in my step, chest out, shoulders back and down, head held high, and a feeling of self-satisfaction connected, if indistinctly, to the realization I was doing this only for myself. I heard this very faint murmur in my head: "John, aren't you glad you came back?" I wasn't completely sure, although I was in a different place than after the first session.

And there was something compelling about Joe that I couldn't identify. He watched me carefully as I left.

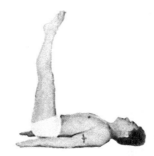

CHAPTER 2

Learning the Ropes

Soon I was going to Joe's gym two times a week without fail. And I was enjoying a great deal of attention from Joe. I came early in the morning, and hardly anyone else showed up to divert his focus from me. The few people who dropped in that early mostly knew the routine. Now and then Joe would say something to them, suggest a correction or slightly change or augment their routine. It wasn't until much later, when I had the routine down pat, that I would come in the afternoon and frequently encounter a full gym.

At the beginning, it would have been easy for me to think that my five-dollar fee entitled me to have Joe at my side always, telling me what to do. No one told me that Joe's instructions were like the "Quick Start" flyer that comes with your smartphone: only just enough to get you started. Neither he nor anyone else explained anything, perhaps because this was something you did and not just something you thought about or tried to understand. I don't recall how or when I knew I was not entitled to receive Joe's full attention. Perhaps someone came in who needed a lot of supervision, and Joe bounced back and forth between the two of us. Or maybe I saw the opposite: someone came in and went through the entire routine without any contact with Joe. Eventually I got the message it was necessary to be able to do the routine by yourself. While that may seem difficult, it really isn't. The routine teaches itself to you.

Positioning myself on the Reformer exactly where Joe told me at the start of the second session mattered. The precise choreography of Joe's program flowed from the correct start. The beginning movement cued your body for the next move, and so on—like a piano player in a bar who can play, on request, thousands of songs without sheet music. Tell the piano player the name of the song, hum a note or two, and his or her hands are flying on the keyboard. There is a chain reaction in the nervous system reconstructing the song note by note, bypassing the conscious memory. So, too, with Joe's choreography.

By withholding instruction and waiting patiently when I got stuck before giving me a hint or cue, Joe forced me to unconsciously tap into this remarkable facility of the body to reconstruct a series of actions. During the early days, my ability to replicate a series of exercises was limited to a chain of three or four movements, but session by session, I was improving without giving it too much thought. This was not how I had learned engineering, or law, or just about everything from the seventh grade on. But it was a lot of fun letting my body surprise me with how much it was picking up.

Even as Joe was withdrawing his attention, I nevertheless felt his presence. He continued to treat me, so I thought, as a favorite pupil. I seemed to get a larger share of his time than anyone else. Maybe because I was the first new student in some time. Maybe there was something else capturing his interest in me. And, even if he wasn't in the gym when I came in, he always showed up as I left the locker room. Other than my concentration and my regularity, I don't know what interested him. I wasn't a dancer like many of his other clients; nothing in my body seemed broken; I wasn't there to look better or to get a daily feel-good workout or learn his method to teach it. Yet I took it very seriously. Joe, with his finely tuned antenna for people's motivations, had to sense something about me that caused him to carefully watch me as I struggled with his program. And I certainly enjoyed his attention.

It's hard to tell when something changes from a frequent activity to a habit, something you schedule much of your life around. I started with a twice a week routine. There were no appointments at Joe's gym. There wasn't even a way to make appointments; there was no appointment book and no phone in the gym. Clara usually answered the phone in their apartment next door if she was there, but that was far from a sure thing. However, I knew if I showed up at seven o'clock on Monday and Thursday mornings, Joe would be there. I could even be a little late since officially it was not an appointment. And he could be late—once I was able to start and do more and more of the routine by myself. This regular rendezvous was only a mutual expectation, but on my calendar I had two private sessions with Joe every week for five dollars each. That was priceless.

And when Joe wasn't there or was occupied with others, Clara was most often present. She didn't take over like Joe did. She stood in the background and watched and listened. It was a different, but no less beneficial, experience. To the extent Joe said little, Clara said even less. To the extent Joe stood over me and watched every little thing, Clara kept a distance. But Clara had an uncanny ability to detect that you were out of position, or not centered, or doing something incorrectly, or stuck not knowing what to do next. She would sense you were in some difficulty by the sound of the machine not sliding smoothly or you breathing in or out at the wrong time, and then she was at your side in a flash, politely, even sweetly, telling you exactly what you needed to know.

Clara and Joe were teammates and had been working together for forty years. Joe was the quarterback; Clara blocked for him. The gym and everything in it and everything that was done in it were Joe's creation. He had designed, built, tested, and maintained every piece of exercise equipment. Neither I nor anyone I knew ever saw Clara do an exercise. But she knew them perfectly. Perhaps Joe had trained her in earlier times. It is hard to imagine he did not. And maybe Clara snuck into the studio at night and worked out. She pitched in seamlessly when it got crowded. She took over when Joe was out. She did it in such a way you didn't miss Joe. It was often a relief getting Clara, particularly when I was tired. Everyone loved Clara. No one felt short-changed when she supervised them.

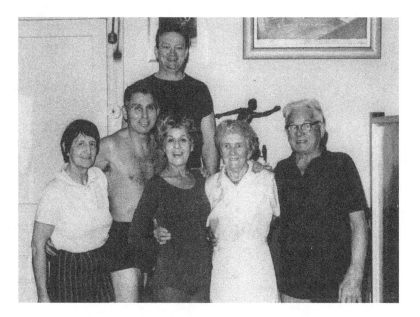

From left: Hannah Sakamirda, Arthur Steel, Bob
Seed, Ruth Steel, Clara and Joe Pilates.

My ability to do the exercise routine slowly but continuously improved from session to session. I was getting stronger, I was moving better, and my posture was improving. I was enjoying the feeling of well-being. I had only to show up at the gym, get down on the Reformer, and clear my mind so I could direct every bit of my attention to moving the right part of my body in the right way at the right time using the right muscles. I learned to quickly transition from one exercise to the next. As I progressed, Joe would add variations on the existing exercises. The first requirement, for everyone, was to master the basic routine.

The progress I made could not be measured. There was no begin-
ner, intermediate, or advanced classification. I couldn't gauge my progress in comparison to anyone else in the gym simply because there
was no standard. The focus was all on the doing and not on competing, even with yourself. There were no objective goals such as do more
exercises, or move faster, or use more resistance. Progress was felt, not
measured. I wasn't there to lose weight, to build killer abs, to reshape
some part of my body. For me, not having any way to measure myself
against others and not having a goal had untethered me from a lifelong
way of being—an affliction, really. Just working through the exercises
without strain, without pushing myself, was enough.

Joe's approach to his exercises and his clients infected everyone's
attitude. People felt privileged to be in his gym, in his presence. Joe
was not just providing a gym in which you could exercise. Nor was he
showing you how to use the equipment or even teaching you a series
of exercises. He was trying to help you learn and acquire exercise,
his particular exercise routine, as a habit to improve your life. His
was not a business; it was a calling, a helping art. Joe's seriousness,
enthusiasm, energy, and insistence on following very strict standards
of conduct in the gym pervaded everything. You were there to learn,
not to work out.

One early morning, I was on the Reformer when there was a knock
at the door. Joe opened it, and a well-dressed and attractive woman
introduced herself as a friend of so-and-so. Joe said: "Nice to meet you,
why are you here?" The well-dressed lady said she was there to get
rid of a bulge in her lower abdomen. Joe said: "We don't do that here,
goodbye." He turned around, closed the door, and left her standing
there. The lady kept talking through the door, in stunned disbelief,
pressing her case for admittance by trying to tell Joe that she "had
made an appointment with Mrs. Pilates and had to get up early to keep
it." Joe just ignored her and returned to instructing me.

Days later, there I was as usual on the Reformer when the well-
dressed lady reappeared. She knocked on the door, as before, and Joe
opened it. I could hear everything. Joe, acting, as if he never had seen
her before, or forgetting he had—I couldn't tell—repeated his question:

"Why are you here?" She replied: "I want to learn your method of exercise." He said "Welcome, come in."

Joe was looking for dedication. He needed you to want to do the work because he knew he could not make you want to do it. Horse to water kind of thing. If he detected that you were serious, that you would commit to the effort, he was with you all the way. All he wanted was for you to keep at it, with some concentration and enthusiasm. And his response was in direct proportion to your commitment.

No matter how athletic or well-coordinated you were, whether you were a dancer, or a gymnast, a boxer, football player, wrestler, golfer, or even a couch potato, you were out of your element when you exercised on his very strange contraptions. He wanted you that way. It was his version of Marine boot camp. Joe's routine was the great leveler, putting all those who came through the door at the same starting place: confused, off balance, perplexed, and a bit desperate trying to figure out what to do. As Joe told each person: "There was no athlete who could do my ten top exercises properly the first time." Well, of course they couldn't, if only because these were unfamiliar movements executed on bizarre equipment.

Despite the strangeness, maybe because of it, there was something rewarding, pleasurable even, that right away attracted a self-selected cross-section of people. The selection process started by the difficulty of getting to Joe. Next the applicant had to pass a mini audition. Not everyone who got past Joe to a Reformer returned.

Joe made it difficult, which I think was because he thought it was easy. Joe believed that exposing anyone to his routine would convince them of the necessity of doing Contrology. He even thought reading his book would be enough. He couldn't accept that everyone wasn't doing Contrology. Yet Joe never understood that his introduction, the peculiar exercises and bizarre equipment, restricted his program to a narrow group. He blamed the absence of demand on the shortsightedness of people, their lack of understanding that Contrology was essential and not optional. He didn't realize, and perhaps didn't care, that his business wasn't thriving because his intake method, akin to throwing a non-swimmer off a boat into deep water, turned potential customers away. He only saw that some people got through the process and got hooked, just like me. Those that lasted and returned regularly had to be magnetically attracted to a program of exercise that was not easy, not convenient, and frequently not comfortable. And they had to overcome an "unwelcome" welcome.

After my first few sessions, the anxiety I had going to Joe's gym vanished. It became a pleasure. For an hour two or three times a week, I was off the treadmill of competition, argument, negotiation, deadlines, concern for others. Going to the gym did require that I push myself during the exercises and concentrate on what I was doing. But these were requirements for which I volunteered. I wasn't working for a client or a senior partner. It was my time, and it cleared my mind.

There were other aspects of Joe's gym that unwound me. A pleasurable relief came with the sudden realization that the only thing I could or needed to control there was myself. Joe controlled everything else: every move you made, the lighting, whether the windows were open. He made all the rules for everyone's conduct and enforced them. So just controlling myself was simple. I knew what I had to do.

Over the years I got to know many of Joe's clients, particularly the nondancers. I was in that gym sweating it out with a lot of type As. I was not alone being attracted to an activity that diverted everyone's attention from their daily lives. By and large, the Pilates addicts were active, even hyperactive, New Yorkers. They were on the go throughout the day and into the night. Getting to the gym, working on themselves in this very noncompetitive atmosphere, was their time away from the hustle and bustle of seeking success or surviving.

As important as the pleasure of self-indulgence was, we also felt the draw of just plain feeling really good, not only right after a session but for hours, even days. It wasn't simply a physical feeling of well-being from exercise. My emotions and my mind seemed to get a cleansing. This was addictive.

Thinking of cleansing, that, too, was part of the gestalt of Contrology. Personal cleanliness was, for Joe, vital. And the shower was the mecca for that virtue. You had to take a shower before you left. Seems obvious; just a matter of hygiene. And, in the summer, with

New York heat and humidity, and no air-conditioning, the shower was essential. But, like so much else with Joe, the shower was not only a way to get clean or get cool. It was a big deal. It was a skin stimulant. It had to be done one way—his way.

Start by visualizing the facility. The men's and ladies' locker rooms were identical. They were approximately four feet wide and eight feet deep, about the size of a medium bathroom. The shower was at the far end, which wasn't very far. And the men's shower was back-to-back with the women's shower. The two showers were the partition between the locker rooms. The showers were the prefab kind, all metal in the days before plastic and fiberglass, the entrance hung with a plastic shower curtain in a striking floral pattern. In each shower was a large bar of brown industrial-strength soap and a ferocious-looking wooden-handled bristle brush. The kind of brush you see Cinderella using to scrub the kitchen floor after the clock struck midnight. Now of course you could bring your own soap, and shampoo, and a soft brush or washcloth. Except for one thing—Joe checked up on you whether you were male or female. He snooped. If he smelled standard soap or shampoo, he just barged in and said, "Use the good soap and brush, your skin is as important as your muscles. It must be clean to breathe." And out he went.

A short time after I started with Joe, I was showering when suddenly the curtain was pulled back and there he was in front of me. Fortunately, I was using the industrial soap; unfortunately, I was not using the brush. Joe stepped right into the shower, dressed in his skimpy shorts and canvas shoes. He wasn't concerned about getting wet nor did he seem to have any notion about my privacy. He grabbed the brush and began soaping it. "Here is how you do it . . ." And he proceeded to scrub me as if I were a piece of outdoor furniture. Up and down, back and forth, bristles getting in the crevices and cracks and making lather like mad. It was uncomfortable. I was red as a beet and exfoliated (a word not then in anyone's vocabulary) near to the point of bleeding. When done, he put the brush down and walked out without another word. I never got scrubbed again, but now and then he opened the shower curtain to check on me, so I became and still am a brush guy, even though I don't use the industrial-strength, commercial-grade model found in every janitorial closet.

Most everyone, at one time or another, had the same experience. And that included women. Because the showers were back-to-back, you could hear very clearly what was going on in the other one. Usually it was just the water running and the typical sounds of someone taking a shower. Not much different from a neighbor showering in most motels. One morning, I had worked out with another fairly new student, a lady somewhat older than I was, maybe forty. I was getting dressed to leave when all of a sudden, I heard a scream from the ladies' shower. Then I heard Joe say, "It is all right, I just need to show you how to take a shower and improve your skin." She said okay, and from what I could hear, or imagine, Joe gave her the very same scrub he gave me. He finished and walked out. I left before the lady. I wondered what she thought. Did she tell anyone?

Many years later, over drinks during a Pilates convention, a former student who was highly respected as one of the few "first generation" instructors told me the story of her "shower lesson." Joe walked in without so much as an "I beg your pardon," scrubbed the hell out of her, and, when she was dressed and leaving, said to her: "You need to work on your breasts. They are too small for your body. You will be much sexier and feel better about yourself with bigger breasts. My exercises will help but drink more milk and eat a little more fat." The woman took it as good and sincere advice, and as she told me she never thought it was anything more than that.

Where did Joe get the nerve to just pop into anyone's shower and give them a scrub? And to disparage a woman's breasts? Did he have advice for men with extra-small or extra-large penises? In talking with Joe over the years, I came to understand that he had a very mechanistic view of the human body. The body, to him, was a special machine. It had life. Just like a mechanical machine, it required maintenance and had to be used properly. Its various parts had to work perfectly together. Joe, of course, did not know about computers where you enter a command in computer language and the machine executes the order. Nor was the body a mechanical device that operated through levers, pulleys, cables, pistons, and the like. The body was trainable. It had a mind. And like any good machine of that day, it had to be oiled and cared for. That was what the shower was all about. You needed to scrub the rust off. Now that scrub has been replaced with fancy technology like laser peels, chemical peels, certain kinds of radiation, and a zillion skin-care products. But really, Joe with his industrial bristle brush was exfoliating everything possible from your skin. All the fancy technology does is to rid the skin of dead cells and open pores. Joe got rid of dead cells with his brush. And undoubtedly a good many live ones as well. Whether pores stayed open under his assault, I don't know.

Though I never saw Joe in the shower, I am sure he scrubbed himself until he was nearly translucent. And poor Clara, if Joe jumped into her shower. She was already a thin little creature with barely enough skin to go around. One good scrub from Joe had to leave her on the edge of survival. No wonder they never had any children. But they had great skin.

***

For years and years, I thought that my nearly instant attraction to a regime of exercise that made me vomit the first time I tried it was so crazy it had to be mine alone. Why I liked it remained a puzzle about which I rarely thought. I never talked to Joe or Clara about what it was that attracted me because to them my interest and enthusiasm were to be expected. There were others in the gym who were dedicated and consistent, and I just assumed that they had their reasons, which differed from mine.

My stiff neck, which brought me to Joe, like a broken car to a mechanic, was never mentioned and vanished from my thoughts. Contrology took care of it. It was as if I had a wart removed from my nose. Contrology still heals my old bones and gets me to the studio even on bad days.

A bedrock of Joe's reputation and his business was his skill—a talent, really—at healing injury. His uncanny instinct led him to the source of the problem, which he corrected with Contrology augmented by specific exercises. He would listen to your complaint impatiently, put you on the Cadillac or the Reformer, have you move as directed, and then, without a word, without a diagnosis, without touching you, ask you to do a few more movements. Then he would tell you what to do at home, and that was it. Not a word about what was wrong and the complete absence of anything resembling a Latin anatomical term.

After only a few weeks with Joe, I strained my back on a Sunday. I was scheduled to fly to Houston the next day. I showed up at Joe's door first thing on Monday, bent over and in pain, just hoping for a quick fix before going to the airport. Looking like the Hunchback of Notre Dame at my Houston meeting was not the impression I needed to make. Joe told me to lie down on the mat, even though I was fully dressed. He put me in position to roll back and forth—the exercise called "Rolling Like a Ball." And he said: "Roll." It hurt. He said "Roll" again. He said, "Get up." My back hurt worse. He said: "Roll on the hotel floor when you get there. Roll before you go to sleep. Tomorrow you will be much better. Have a good trip."

He was right. The next day I was fine.

Looking back fifty years, I now know what drew me to return that second day. True, there is a mysterious magnetic force at the heart of Pilates. And true, almost any form of exercise that you can squeeze into an otherwise busy workday makes you feel better, even virtuous. These attractions were certainly a part of what kept me at it after the first resistance wore off. However, I believe the real reason I not only kept doing Pilates but worked very hard to perpetuate it after Joe was gone was something from my family dynamic. Unconsciously, I was in search of Pilates while at the same time Joe was unconsciously looking for me.

I was raised in an upper-middle-class household. On paper, I had an ideal childhood. My parents were happily married, never fought, in fact, never raised their voices. We lived very comfortably in nice places, and my brother and I were well cared for and constantly attended to. I learned good manners and proper behavior. And how to study and get good grades and be competitive. I did well in everything I engaged in and even survived the strict rigors of Culver Military Academy in Indiana, which for a thirteen-year-old Jewish kid from a New York City public school was no small feat. In fact, once I learned the ropes of military school life at Culver (which was not optional—sink or swim), I did exceptionally well and was accepted into Princeton University. My parents pushed us, encouraged us to excel, monitored our progress, and urged us on. When we got to the top of whatever figurative mountain we were directed to climb, there was always another mountain. The only thing that was missing from my constant efforts to push myself was parental approval: no small thing. A simple "I know that was hard, and I am proud of you" might have done the trick. Just an occasional pat on the back would have been sufficient. But the expressions "attaboy," "good job," "well done," or even "I'm proud of you" were neither in my parents' vocabulary nor in their body language.

When I went to meet Joe, exercising was just another mountain. I was pushed there by my mother. Once I survived that first lesson, though, there was a difference. My continuation was optional. It would have been easy for me to say that it was not for me and didn't help my neck, or that he was a quack or make some other excuse. But unconsciously, I sensed I could get the appreciation I needed from Joe Pilates. Joe was no better at verbalizing approval than my parents, nor was he physically demonstrative. He didn't give out pats on the back. Yet he transmitted that he genuinely approved of my efforts. It came through his touch, his enthusiasm, his complete focus on me. He let me know without words that he appreciated how hard I was working, and that was enough. He was the dream coach: he made me want to try harder by making me feel good. He made me chase those good feelings of accomplishment by accomplishing more. And the more I sensed that he saw what I accomplished, the better I felt. I desperately needed someone to acknowledge that I was giving it my all.

I couldn't get a grip on my life in 1963. I know I wasn't the only twenty-eight-year-old who had followed a prescribed route and suddenly found himself veering off the map. I imagined a cartoonist's bubble of small text in the margin of the map: "Pal, you are on your own from here on out." I had followed all the instructions given to me, never knowing or having been told the destination, and I was not sure of where I was or where I was headed. I was married at twenty-eight for the second time, just back from Reno, Nevada, where I went to get untangled from Wife Number One. I had a child on the way and was starting a new job at a small law firm. I had no idea why I was married for the second time instead of being a carefree bachelor. I liked my job and my fellow workers but worried that I didn't have the aggression or the motivation to succeed in this desperately competitive environment. My New York social life was also a competitive jungle—everyone trying to outdo everyone else by making more money or knowing the right people or being big shots or having a better house, apartment, car, wardrobe. I didn't fit in because I didn't like this kind of competition and was not good at it. More daunting was the fear of failure. I preferred to stand aside and take a righteous position decrying money grubbing and social climbing. So here I was stuck in a business and social world that I couldn't stand and from which I could see no escape. Like every fool wandering around in a snowstorm, I was looking for some sign of where to go, just to find myself.

My inner compass pointed to Joe as someone who could head me in the right direction by simply acknowledging my worth—as odd as that may sound about a man who never said "attaboy" or "good job." But after our first encounter, he did make it clear he wanted me back in two days at seven in the morning. And I felt his undivided attention and even got a strong sense that he enjoyed helping me because of my response. I didn't *know* what I may have been seeking after that first session, or even during the rest of Joe's life, but I never stopped feeling it.

I know it now. His hand is still on my back fifty-three years later. And his arthritic finger is pointing up and onward.

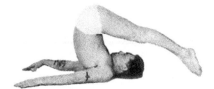

CHAPTER 3

Joe and Clara Off Duty

One day about six months after I started with Joe, Clara stopped me as I was leaving the gym. "What do you do after work?" she asked.

Clara and I had not exchanged more than a hello or a few corrections to my exercises since the day we met. I thought the question a bit strange, inquiring into something unrelated to the gym. I assumed it was somehow health related. After all, she was dressed like a nurse. I told her I usually went out with a few junior lawyers, paralegals, and secretaries to the bar across the street to grab a beer.

"Would you like to come back to our apartment sometime and have a beer with Joe?" she asked. "Joe would really enjoy that."

I said okay. We settled on the next night at seven thirty.

Going to Joe and Clara's apartment was quite a change from my after-office routine in the saloon with my coworkers. There we'd complain about our clients, or the lawyer on the other side, or a judge, or our boss, or life in general. If I didn't go back to the office or wasn't meeting my wife or friends for dinner, I usually walked home, sometimes grabbing a hamburger on the way.

But I was in no hurry to get home because I wasn't happy at home. Whether Joe or Clara knew about my home life, I had no idea, but I suspected Joe, with his ability to read muscles and movements, sensed tension in my body. He had never mentioned anything.

That meek, shy Clara had been delegated to make the invitation told me something about Joe. Right off I knew I was the subject of some discussion in the Pilates household. Most surprising, however, was the thought that this blustery, autocratic man, seemingly in total control of everything in his world, didn't ask me himself. I presumed he was either quite shy or truly afraid of rejection. The alternative, that it was the European way to have the woman of the house do the inviting, never occurred to me. My curiosity was piqued by what seemed like urgency.

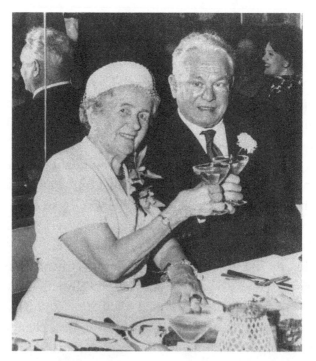

Joe and Clara off duty on Joe's eightieth birthday, 1963.

Joe and Clara lived next door to the gym; the proximity was no accident. Their life was the gym and they went between the two spaces like others might go between the kitchen and the living room. The building was nineteenth century, poorly maintained, and very worn. This was New York in the 1960s—prosperous, striving to be modern—and here were these elderly, far from modern people, living in the same apartment for almost forty years. Perhaps some found it charming, reminiscent of Europe.

I showed up at the appointed hour and was suddenly in the inner sanctum of the Pilates family. Clara, who was at the door with Joe when I entered, went through a curtained entry to my left, and I heard a refrigerator door open and close. She returned with two bottles of beer and handed them to Joe and me wordlessly. As much of a surprise as the gym was when I first saw it, the apartment was even more unexpected. The thing that hit me right off was how dark it was, almost like a movie theater. I saw lamps about, but they must have had five-watt refrigerator bulbs in them, just enough light to navigate by. The apartment was one large room divided by flimsy walls that went up about eight feet but didn't reach the ceiling. In New York real estate ads, it would be described as a "large, comfortable studio"—a glamorizing NY stretch for these digs. It took me a minute or two for my eyes to adjust even from the dark hall. There in front of me was a wood table on solid wood legs, surrounded by, of all things, six of the exact same exercise devices—called "the Wunda Chair"—as in the gym.

By flipping the chair on its back and making one other minor adjustment, the exercise apparatus nicely doubled as furniture—a dining chair. I would later learn that the transition from exercise apparatus to dining chair took about five seconds and required no tools.

The Wunda Chair is an excellent example of Joe's design aesthetic, perhaps even his philosophy of life. He started, focused on the exercise potential of a piece of equipment, and then tried to make it into a piece of household furniture. This dual-purpose design—exercise equipment / household furniture—was applied to other equipment, which I will get to shortly. The Wunda Chairs are still built almost exactly as Joe made them, although while I see them in studios, I have never seen them in anyone's dining room.

Below is the nicely upholstered chair, with cushions for the back and seat. The one on the right is the exercise version made by Balanced Body. It is the same chair flipped on its back (down to the left) with the seat and back cushions removed. Joe called it the Wunda Chair, and that it surely was.

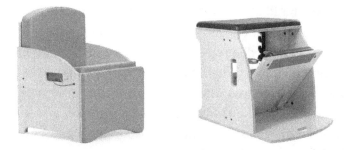

Wunda Chair transformed.

Joe also made a Universal Reformer model with an upholstered top, turning the exercise equipment into a chaise with an intriguing ergonomic shape.

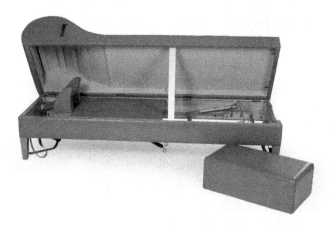

Joe's Reformer/chaise lounge.

Glancing to the right were what appeared to be two metal bunk beds. I knew they were beds only because they had the dimensions of a bed and included pillows, sheets, and blankets tightly made up like army bunks. At each corner of the first bed, extending up about six feet, were four ordinary galvanized steel pipes, all interconnected at the top to a rectangle of horizontal pipes. A plumber's version of a Louis XIV four-poster bed. Hanging from the horizontal pipes at the top, at the pillow end, were several springs, a small trapeze, some slings and straps, and something made of sheepskin. The other bed had the same superstructure but no dangling equipment. All the hanging gear on the far bed was familiar from the gym, but its presence on a bed was incongruous. Glancing from the chairs to the bed, I realized that Clara and Joe's apartment was more Joe's laboratory than it was a home. The thought that I might have been there as a lab rat crossed my mind.

Joe and I sat down across from each other on the aforementioned Wunda Chairs, while Clara, in her nurse's uniform, stood behind and to the side of Joe. They looked very formal and stiff, like a very old photograph where one person was seated, the other standing, and both holding their breath to avoid any motion. This tableau served to accentuate the huge cultural, never mind age, differences between the third generation Ivy League–educated guy in the suit and tie, and the immigrant Joe in his gym shorts and Clara in her nurse's outfit. Joe thanked me for coming and hoped he had not inconvenienced me. I was uncomfortable in this very strange environment. He and Clara were more so. This was not the gym next door where Joe was in control, the cock of the walk, with the program laid out and fully understood. Conversation started very slowly.

"What do you do for a living?" Joe asked, after we both had a few swigs of beer.

I said, "I am a lawyer, frequently in court." I expected more questions on that topic, such as Did I like it? Or what kind of cases? But instead he went to more questions about my life. "Are you married?" "Do you have children?" "Where do you live?" followed in short order.

After I answered, he asked, digging deeper, "Why doesn't your wife come to my gym? Your mother and father do."

All I could say to that one was she wasn't interested in doing exercises and didn't get along with my mother or father. I left out that she didn't get along with me either.

The conversation was slow, stiff, and very heavy. I was defensive and not at all prepared to open a window on my home life. I was the same guarded self with them that I was with everyone, but here I had the sense that my cover-up wasn't working too well.

When the preliminaries had run their course, Joe motioned me over to one of the beds, the one with the contraptions hanging from the overhead pipes. He had resumed his role as physical trainer. He said, "Lie down." My paranoia about being a lab rat popped back into my head, but, like on day one, I was trapped. Then he told me to grab the handle on the right side next to the mattress and push it down and away. I pushed it as directed. And wonder of wonders, the bed split down the middle lengthwise, and the center smoothly dropped eight or ten inches. For a second it was scary. The bed had a trapdoor that mercifully didn't open all the way and drop me on the floor. But I was Joe's lab rat without question. There I was on my back, on his bed, lying in a V caused by the mattress sagging without support down its length, waiting for the mattress with me on board to slip through the crack and dump me on the floor.

But the mattress held, and more instructions came from Joe: "Put your hands behind your head, relax your elbows down to the bed, put your heels together, and separate your knees to each side of the bed."

I was back under his total control as if he had just hypnotized me. What followed was precisely what a hypnotist might say, only with a pronounced German accent: "Now you are comfortable in the position of total support, total relaxation. That is how you should sleep. You would need less. And when you wake up, you do some of the exercises for fifteen minutes using the springs hanging from the bed. Then you are ready for your day ahead."

I confirmed to him that the bed was incredibly comfortable, and quipped, "If every bed was split in the middle, procreation would be exceptionally difficult, and humans would eventually disappear."

He replied with an annoyed tone, "Only those people who could learn to procreate in my bed, or in a hammock, should survive. Nobody else." He added that sex in the split bed was better. "More relaxing to the person underneath." Basic Darwinism à la Joe.

When instructed, I pulled up the lever, with some effort, lifting me and restoring the mattress back to being flat. A necessary step to get out of this contraption. I got up, and Joe proceeded to show me the inner workings of his bizarre invention.

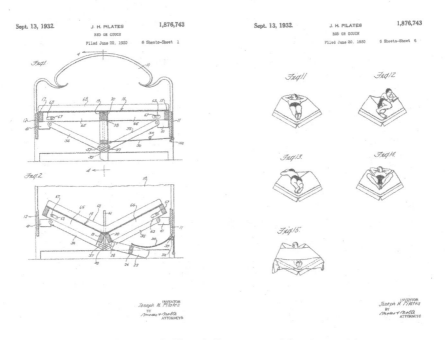

Joe's V-Bed patent (left) and illustration of sleeping positions.

Picture a very simple bedspring—a metal rectangle crisscrossed by metal straps attached to the rectangle with short, coiled springs. It was a bouncy base for a thin mattress. Joe had cut the crisscrossed straps lengthwise down the middle and added an inner metal frame on each side, resulting in two side-by-side bedsprings in the frame. To hold these two segments up, and to prevent them from opening all the way and dropping the occupant on the floor, which was my fear, he'd put a substantial metal roller below the added lengthwise frame elements in the middle. The roller operated through the handle I pushed down or pulled up, either bringing the springs up to level or allowing them to open and drop down. Very simple, primitive really, a bit squeaky, requiring a good tug to get things back to flat and certainly introducing a mechanical element into what for centuries has been unmechanized.

Once, many years later, I found myself in a high-tech hospital bed after hip replacement surgery. The doctor had ordered my legs raised, while my upper body remained flat. I was uncomfortable despite a very fine drug cocktail. The nurse had me put my hands behind my head and placed a pillow under my elbows. Then he put a pillow under each side of my buttocks. The nurse said that this V configuration was a more natural position for the hip joint and that it was more relaxing for all the muscles. Suddenly recalling Joe's bed and the V effect, I told the nurse that is exactly what Joe Pilates would have done. He was perplexed and he asked, "Joe who?" I told him. He must have asked around at the nurses' station, because after that I had nurses visiting me constantly to ask about Joe Pilates. It turned out many in the nursing staff took Pilates classes right in the hospital, where a teacher came every day. My nurse had placed me in a position like the one in which I had ended up in Joe's dropped-center bed—convincing me that, once again, Joe had been way ahead of his time.

After the bed demonstration, it was time to go. I thanked them, and Clara asked when I could come again, sweetening the invitation with: "I'll make soup next time." I had to give a return trip some thought. Like my first exercise session with Joe, this first social visit was not fun. It resembled, at least in my imagination, a first visit with a somewhat distant relative who lived in a different country and spoke poor English, my only language. Despite seeing Joe for two or three hours every week for the past six months, we were strangers outside of the gym.

Moreover, I couldn't understand why Joe and Clara wanted me back, since they were not any more at ease than I had been. Yet again I felt this little emotional battle raging between an undefined attraction or need on my part, and my dislike of uncomfortable situations like this one. Could it be that just because they wanted me back was enough for me? Or perhaps I didn't want to trifle with my teacher-student relationship by rejecting them? I was conflicted and not happy about it. This sudden push for social contact felt strange to me. After all, I was twenty-eight, and Joe and Clara were both over eighty.

But once again, my instinctive reflex overpowered my brain. I quickly replied, "How about next week, same time?" Clara said, "Okay," and that was that.

After that, I showed up at Joe and Clara's nearly every week. Sometimes it was just for a beer, sometimes I brought in pizza, but most of the time Clara had soup on their hot plate. The soup was good. She made stock and used bones to do so. Then she added some carrots, beans, and usually some sausage or frankfurters. That with a few slices of dark bread, preceded by a beer or two, was their usual fare, and I was happy to share it. Even after Joe's death in 1967, I continued to visit Clara once or twice a week until her death in 1976.

***

The Joe in his apartment was different from the Joe in the gym. The clients who attended his gym knew him as a physical trainer. As such, he was something of a celebrity, like a symphony conductor on the podium. His presence alone directed the performance of the various activities on the floor. Like a conductor, he kept the studio hopping while working with a client. Whether as the "maestro" or your personal trainer, he remained distant. Nothing intimate or even friendly crossed that relationship divide.

Some people, dancers mostly, knew him as a savior—the person who kept them dancing, or stopped their back pain, or put a zip in their step, or some other career enhancing or enabling therapy. He helped professional golfers eliminate pain in their swing; he helped hairdressers and barbers work pain-free all day with their arms raised. He improved singers' breath control. As the person who worked his obscure magic to solve a physical problem that ofttimes doctors, chiropractors, or massage therapists couldn't, he was a medicine man. Someone who worked miracles.

Joe had part-time assistants who seemed to appear from nowhere at busy times. They all knew the routines, were very helpful, but remained very much in his shadow. Even though Joe may have had different relationships with some of them or thought some of them better at following his program, or better with his clients, he treated them the same way he treated us, his clients. That is, he let them do what they believed necessary and never publicly corrected them. Perhaps he gave looks, or made small gestures, but I never saw him speak to his assistants. Managing the staff was, I suspect, Clara's responsibility. His assistants seemed to know, as if by instinct, what was expected of them. One of the women assistants was reputed to be his mistress, but even the most perceptive prognosticator of an intimate relationship would not have been able to detect that.

To Clara, Joe was her devoted mate, her protector, and the sun rose and set on him. Clara assisted in and managed the gym, and she was treated there like all other assistants. She was Joe's entire family. He had no contact with the family he left behind in Germany, little with his brother in Saint Louis. Who knows what the children and stepchild he left behind in Germany or his brother and sister-in-law thought of him? He appeared to have no interest in or connection to any members of the Pilates family, although his niece had worked as an assistant in the studio long before my time. His only other social connections that I knew about were as a member of a Masonic lodge, and his brethren there saw a side of him unknown to others. There he drank beer and spoke German. At the Lodge he was just one of the immigrants getting on in New York.

On the few occasions when I was in a social situation with Joe, he was very quiet. He never mentioned any of his illustrious clients or spoke as a Contrology evangelist. Before my time, a group of his clients had tried to organize a foundation to perpetuate his work. To them, he had been the most difficult, frustrating person they had ever dealt with. One of them, a doctor, told me that the more they tried to help him organize his business and devise a succession strategy, the more he resisted them. He would sit quietly at meetings, then suddenly interrupt everything and shout, "You are trying to steal my work while I am still here!" Then he would storm out.

In the gym, Joe seemed to me partly like a college professor with a huge reputation who entered the lecture room, gave his lecture without interacting with the students, and left, usually to applause. The other part was a surgeon who visited the patient before an operation and tried to be friendly and personal but was emotionally detached . . . just there to fix a body. There was nothing personal or familiar in his relationships inside the gym. His clients and assistants were strictly about learning, doing, or teaching Contrology. He rarely knew his clients' names, and if he did, he didn't use them.

Despite the emotional distance, though, Joe dealt with his clients with professional dedication. He was a hands-on instructor: he poked where he thought a poke would help, he pushed where the client needed a little extra stretch, and he touched people wherever he decided they needed to feel something rather than hear it. He conveyed a great deal of information and warmth through his hands. I never heard one complaint or objection to any of his touching.

My social contact gave me a broader and different perspective. By coming to the apartment and sitting through what was always a stiff conversation with Joe and Clara, I saw them in an unusual light. My social relationship to them was peculiar and hard to put in any known category. I was certainly not a friend, nor was I their attorney. The relationship felt slightly familial, as if it was obligatory. How or why I felt obligated, I have never understood.

The closest I can come to defining the family-like relationship with Joe was grandfather–grandson. I did not see Joe as a grandfather, nor was I in search of one, as I had a perfectly good one. My guess is that Joe needed someone to perpetuate his legacy, and a grandson-like person might fill the bill. Or maybe he just wanted a grandson. Joe and Clara did not have children. Joe may have had real grandchildren back in Germany whom he may not have known about. He never mentioned the family left behind. Maybe as he got older, he felt bad about them. And there I was, old enough to no longer be a bother and young enough to be a grandson. I was conscripted.

Joe was not particularly good at being a grandfather to someone who was essentially a stranger. Nor was I particularly prepared to be his grandchild. Joe was not like any member of my family. I had fond memories of my mother's father, whom I knew only slightly but nevertheless remembered as loving and warm. He died when I was about ten. My father's father died when my dad was thirteen, and my paternal grandmother married a worthy substitute long before I was born. My step-grandfather had no children, and that was a good thing because he didn't like little kids. I spent a good part of my growing-up years living with my step-grandfather and my grandmother, whom I adored. When I got past the so-called difficult years and no longer needed to be played with or read to, my step-grandfather started to tolerate me, then he began to enjoy me. He taught me to ride a bicycle, use tools, and be independent. He took me to California every summer where he had business, and I trailed around after him all day. I sense he wanted to fill gaps in my parenting that he mistakenly thought my father neglected: teaching or lecturing on hard work, resilience, and perseverance. After becoming a lawyer, I was the only family member he trusted, other than my grandmother. My step-grandfather went to the horse racetrack nearly every afternoon, and he took me with him on occasion and tried to teach me how to handicap horses: a skill he was not particularly adept at despite years of avid interest and conscientious practice. I was terrible—you needed to be able to remember the names of horses, jockeys, trainers, and a whole bunch of statistics—not my strong suit.

Occasionally, Joe would ask me if I would like a Saturday morning session. I enjoyed those—the gym was empty, and he was completely focused on me. Afterwards Joe always wanted to take a walk. His favorite destination was the Central Park Zoo, a ten-minute trip. Clara would make some sandwiches and pack them in the cellophane bag from the loaf of bread, and we would head up Eighth Avenue into the park at 59th Street, then over to the zoo and a bench opposite the lion or tiger cages.

Joe was transfixed watching large caged cats. He noticed their every move and was particularly attentive to anything that resembled either exercise or stretching, which is about all they did. Every time an animal made a move that caught his attention, he would tap me on the leg and point it out. He would then tell me why the animal was doing what it was doing, and how he had incorporated that stretch or exercise into Contrology. Watching the tragedy of caged animals was unpleasant for me. Joe, on the other hand, loved to observe an animal's behavior in confined space, and he compared every instinctive move made by the animal to a movement of Contrology. As I watched the animal, I recalled my first impression of Joe as a lion on its hind legs. Except here it was caged. The lion's need to exercise and stretch was what Joe said we city dwellers needed for our survival. I looked across at Joe, and from the intensity on his face, I realized he was watching himself in that enclosure. He knew what it was like to be caged. We would sit there for about an hour and eat the sandwiches, and suddenly, without a word, Joe would get up and start back home.

Even though visiting Joe and Clara became a regular part of my life, our social engagements remained quite stiff for some time. Neither Joe nor Clara had any interest in current events, politics, religion, or any of the cultural stuff New Yorkers feed on. I learned to tolerate long silences. They were comfortable with these silences, but initially I was not. Slurping soup helped. We simply did not have much to talk about. The walks were an improvement. Joe would talk more, and the silence wasn't so deadly.

Joe's past, a topic with great potential, was never touched upon. It was clearly off-limits. Neither Joe nor Clara opened a crack into their past. If I showed any interest in their history, even in the somewhat recent past from the time they arrived in New York, they ignored me without so much as an explanation. I wasn't writing a book, nor was I particularly curious, so it didn't bother me. My step-grandfather, also an immigrant, didn't like to talk about his past either.

Most conversations with Joe turned to the one common subject: how Contrology was the balm for all human ills. At one point I became curious about the origin of Contrology and thought that maybe Joe would be happy to talk about it. The history of Contrology might not disturb the ashes of Joe's personal story. I was wrong. Obviously, Contrology's past and Joe's were linked. When I asked him how he started teaching Contrology, or how he developed it, his answer was always the same: "I understand human anatomy." That was all. It would only be years later that I came to realize just how much Joe had left out of our conversations. Clara was much easier to know. She was far closer to what I perceived as normal. Joe referred to Clara as his wife, and she went by Clara Pilates. But as I'd learn later, there was no record of them ever having been married. That didn't matter: they were married in every sense of the word, with or without state sanction.

While Joe was still alive, my relationship with Clara was different and more distant than the one I had with Joe. Clara was always kind and friendly. But Joe was so dominant during our times together, even when he was mostly silent, that it was impossible to develop a separate relationship with Clara. That changed after Joe's death in 1967, when we grew closer—in many ways our relationship was much closer and more real than the one with Joe. I took care of Clara's legal problems—her business situation with both the continuation of the New York operation and helping others to open Pilates studios with her permission. I made sure she had enough money to live on, and I usually had dinner with her once a week. I could and did talk to her about my life and ask about hers. Concerning hers, she missed Joe terribly, but Clara was truly tough and just carried on as she thought he would have wanted. Clara was very warmed by the thought that several others, including me, were working hard to perpetuate Joe's legacy. And she did try to make sure we respected the work, but with her badly failing eyesight and the infirmity of old age, she had no choice but to let us do it as best we could. When I, or others, would bring her over to the new studio on 56th Street (which we will get to shortly), she would sit in the background and watch. Rarely would she have anything to say. Now and then she would relate to an old client, including my parents, but she seemingly didn't want to interrupt their session. On her ninetieth birthday we had a wonderful party for her, and she was radiant and very happy. But mostly her later years were very lonely.

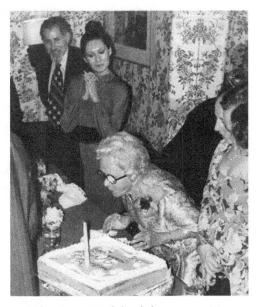

Clara's ninetieth birthday party, 1971.

During earlier times together, there existed a huge gulf between Joe and Clara and me, which was never overcome. What has stayed with me over the years has been my memory of what it felt like to be around both of them—and the fact that I hardly knew anything about either one. Indeed, I think I learned more about Joe from writing this book than I learned from being with him. Back then I made no attempt to separate Joe the man from Joe the teacher and inventor of Contrology. He was, I sadly confess, mostly identified in my mind with the work. Perhaps that is often true of how children see their grandparents. When I look back, I behaved with Joe more like a very young grandchild rather than the self-sufficient professional I was at the time. And, not to put too fine a point on it, maybe playing the part of grandson was the only way I could have related to him.

***

When summer came and the days got longer and warmer, Joe would suggest we take a walk in the evening after the late-afternoon rush was over. Usually we traveled downtown along Eighth Avenue. And that was a sight to behold, I am sure. On the street, Joe looked like a strange old man, wearing nothing more than a pair of skimpy gym shorts over his skinny bowlegs, a white turtleneck long-sleeve cotton shirt covering his barrel chest, and canvas slippers. He was deeply tanned and exceptionally muscular. He'd hook his arm into mine, European-style, somewhat dragging me along: a much younger guy wearing a well-tailored suit, a shirt and tie, and depending on the weather, sometimes a coat. We were a study in contrasts, walking at a very crisp pace. Sometimes Joe would have a pipe in his mouth, and in the bowl, sticking straight up, a cheap cigar. That the lit embers from the upright cigar blew in his face didn't bother him.

Like so much else with Joe Pilates, our walks took a bit of getting used to. He had a glide to his walk with his legs doing the minimum to propel him, but at the same time, he was on the balls of his feet, leaning slightly forward, and swinging the outside arm as if he were running—the other was crossed with mine, and he used it as a pry bar to force me to keep up with him. He moved very energetically and aggressively, yet with hardly any effort. His pace was somewhere between a stroll and a power walk. We closed in on anyone in our path, and when we were behind someone, they sensed it and gave us the space to pass. Even with only one eye and diminished depth perception, nothing seemed to slow Joe down. We'd cut through the human traffic like a motorcycle white-lining it between lanes of slowly moving traffic down the LA freeways.

Eighth Avenue between 42nd Street and 59th Street—where Central Park begins—was a bustling place at the end of the day. The roadway was crowded with cars, buses, cabs, and trucks of all sizes. The sidewalks were also jammed at rush hour—people trying to get home from work or headed somewhere for the evening. Some people were even going *to* work, this being the city that never sleeps. Hungry people, thirsty people, impatient people weaving in and out to get into a faster lane. The drivers were leaning on their horns for no apparent reason other than it was the New York way of communicating. When we had to cross a side street, Joe kept going despite the red traffic light, despite the traffic. Cars simply had to stop for him. I was far too timid to ask him to slow down or to observe the lights. Like Moses at the Red Sea, Joe proceeded, and the rest of New York parted before him.

It was scary at first. I was locked on to his arm but skittering about madly trying to stay in step. After a while I relaxed, fell in with his pace, and ignored the dangers and the occasional rebuke from someone we may have jostled, cut off, or otherwise offended. Joe got yelled at: "Hey old man, where's da fire, pal?" spoken in perfect New Yorkese. He ignored the comments. People stared not only because of Joe's outfit but because man with man, arm-in-arm contact was unusual. With Joe, there was no sense being self-conscious or polite. He wasn't either, and good manners didn't work on a busy New York sidewalk. He adapted to his environment, took his walk, got some exercise and what he thought was fresh air. He kept his preferred pace without bothering anyone, except now and then for only a moment. A lesson I needed.

It was during these walks that Joe would talk, almost always about something related to Contrology. As we walked along, he would correct my walking posture and style. He'd tell me to put my shoulders back "but not up." And my chin down "but not droopy." And, because we were arm in arm, with his hand on my wrist, he fully controlled our pace and forced me to walk evenly. It felt to me like I was on a treadmill having a cardiac stress test.

Not only would he fix my walking posture, but he had comments about everyone who passed by. To Joe, people on New York sidewalks were specimens of bad bodies and bad physical habits. Everyone needed some correction, and Contrology would fix them in a jiffy.

"See that lady over there? She has her head at a tilt and that is because she takes a longer step with one foot which causes her to put that hip forward and that requires her to tilt her head to keep balanced. One day probably already she will have a bad back. And then she will go to a doctor who will tell her that she has a curved spine and sell her a brace and give her a big bill. Two weeks with me on the Reformer and Cadillac and the bad back will be gone and her head will be straight when she walks."

Someone else would come into view, and Joe would say: "That man over there must be a hairdresser or a golfer or a dentist because he swings one arm very loosely and the other one sort of hangs like it's tired out. One day his shoulder will start to get stiff and hurt and he will go to a doctor who will give him some pills which cost money. He will take the pills and the pain will go away for a while. And he will take more pills and his stomach will get bad and who knows what will happen to him. Two weeks in the gym every day he can fix the shoulder learn to swing the arms the same and then just two times a week he stays fine. No doctor no pills no pain. Very easy."

The faster Joe walked, the more animated he became. And the more animated he became, the more he vented. Deep down, Joe was an angry man. He was angry at the world for not recognizing Contrology as a great discovery. He was angry at the medical profession for not seeing Contrology as the most effective medicine. He simply couldn't understand, much less accept, that anybody who professed to know the human body and was committed to caring for it didn't instantly recognize that exercise, and particularly his series of exercises, was the cure-all.

Joe didn't accept that he couldn't change the world. He was convinced he had discovered the fountain of youth and thought that the world would instantly learn of it through some mystical force. But during Joe's life, only very few people would know of Contrology, and I doubt any of them gave up their medical doctor.

Joe, when walking with me, was much more talkative than in his apartment with Clara. While he wasn't inclined to talk about his life, his view of life seeped out. One of the subjects that opened when he was out of earshot of Clara was sex. One afternoon, he spotted a comely woman, perhaps a prostitute, coming at us along Eighth Avenue. "You know, sex is as important as doing Contrology," he said. I remember it distinctly because Joe acknowledging anything to be as important as Contrology was a surprise. He proceeded to elaborate.

"From day one, man had to use his physical being to survive, and from day two had to have sex," he continued. "Now I will tell you my secret. One day I thought that if I could get exercise to be as much fun as sex, everyone would do it a lot. And then the world would be a healthier, happier place. Who would want to go to war when they could stay home and enjoy sex and exercise? Nobody! But no one can get exercise to be as much fun as sex. So, and this is private between us, I made many exercises like movements in sex. That does two things: it tricks the body into moving naturally and fluidly like it is having sex, and it strengthens the right muscles, so it improves their sex life."

I tried not to let this stunning revelation change my pace, but I am sure I faltered. Then I mumbled, trying my best to keep my voice calm and clinical: "So how did you make exercise like sex?"

"Ever since I was a young boxer, I knew a lot about the body and could feel how my muscles worked when I moved, so I designed the exercises to use all my muscles, and stretch them out, and I used movements people do when doing sex. Once they start to enjoy doing my exercises, like you did, wives make their husbands go, like your mother did. Husbands make their wives go, like you should. Contrology improves your performance, your stamina, and the best part, it makes you want sex more—a good thing."

Using "movements people do when doing sex" sounded plausible. I asked when he designed these sexually oriented exercises. He totally ignored me and went on.

"So, Contrology strengthens the body and makes it work good for sex. And sex makes people happy and healthier. There you have some of it. Now I never tell anyone this, but I thought that everyone saw so many sexual positions in the exercises. No one has ever mentioned a word to me about it. No one has ever told me the exercises have improved their sex life. People are shy about their sex lives, so I don't advertise it. They get it unconsciously. Just think about all the exercises."

I was still with Joe, struggling to keep up while totally focused on what I was hearing and experiencing some unease. Joe just kept going. This, I sensed, was wisdom from an elder.

"You, John, just think about the positions of the women you see doing the exercises. For many of the exercises they are on their backs, legs up in the air, spread. You like that position, right? Best thing, they are strengthening their stomachs, but they are learning to control their legs and strengthening the important muscles in their body and in their sex parts. Other times they are sitting up, sometimes straddling the box, pulling their inner thighs in and working their pelvis back and forth. Like they were riding a horse at a slow canter. And look what these exercises do for their breasts."

Joe mentioned the Magic Circle, one of his many little portable devices. It is a circular contraption about a foot in diameter made from strips of steel similar to small barrel hoops, with two hand-sized wood blocks on the circumference opposing each other. To this day it is a very popular device. Joe was on a roll. "I mostly use the Magic Circle for women. I put it between their knees or their ankles and tell them to squeeze. Sometimes, I have them hold it in front of them and squeeze. Now and then they ask me why I named it 'magic' and I tell them because it has a magical effect on their thighs or their breasts. But you want to know the real reason I named it 'magic'? It's because of the magic that happens when they have sex. Their squeeze is so much stronger that now and then their husband says, 'Wow, that was magic.'"

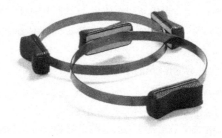

Joe's Magic Circle.

We were moving along quickly, and we were far from the apartment. I thought Joe was going to suggest we turn back and give me some time to think these things over. Turn back we did, but Joe was wound up. "Now, John, think about yourself. Has your sex life improved? Tell me the truth."

Despite my discomfort, I was amazed that Joe had sensed something bothering me that I forced myself not to think or ever talk about.

I hesitated. "My sex life hasn't improved, but not for lack of the proper exercises. And it won't. It was bad before I came to you, and it is still bad. Much in my life has improved, but not my sex life."

"Why is it bad? Your wife has something wrong with her?" he asked.

I explained that my wife and I didn't get along. We had different goals, different ambitions, different values. She didn't like mine and I didn't like hers. I resented her continuous shopping for clothes, her social climbing, her nagging me to get a Mercedes when we didn't even need a car in New York. "And there are lots of things about me she doesn't like. I don't like them either. I drink too much at social events and get obnoxious. I don't take her side when my mother puts her down. She calls me a spoiled mama's boy. I get annoyed when I must take care of things or take care of her. When we do have sex, from my side it is full of anger, from her side it is a commodity I haven't properly paid for. It's terrible!"

This was the first time in my life I had revealed to anyone the most upsetting, and most private, part of my life.

Joe said, "Okay, sex with your wife is no good, so have sex with someone else, feel like a man, feel good, and maybe you won't be so angry and mean toward your wife. You won't be the first guy I know, or even the first woman, who improved their life at home by improving their life outside the home. Most people it helps; some it ruins. But better to find out, than suffer. I hate suffering."

***

Important for me to hear from the person I subconsciously looked to as a savior were the two notions Joe put forth: That it was not only okay to have sex outside marriage, but that if sex at home was no good, then extramarital sex was actually necessary; and two, that there were plenty of women who wanted sex for the fun of it. The latter I knew, but I was hesitant to get involved because I was so worried about how to get uninvolved. With this quasi-medical prescription, my daily routine suddenly shifted. The force impelling me to get to the gym early three mornings a week shifted ever so slightly to picking a time when one of these women who wanted sex for fun might be there. With Joe's blessing, coming from the man who oversaw my body, my life changed, forever.

Sometimes Joe talked about how Contrology also strengthened men's sexual abilities. He referred to the Hundred, a pumping exercise; Coordination, which required you to do one thing with one part of your body and something quite different with another; and Short and Long Spine, which loosened your lumbar area, giving you (as he put it) more powerful thrust, as if we men were hydraulic pistons. Joe said he had never heard of any of his students throwing their back out while having sex or suffering a heart attack like Governor Nelson Rockefeller supposedly had. Joe said that if you can get through a Contrology routine, you are good to go in bed. But he did recommend that horizontal sex was safer for the heart than vertical sex. Just like warming up on the Reformer, lying down was far better for the heart. Who knew that getting on the Reformer to do leg work was foreplay?

I remember another walk when Joe talked about how sex helped your body and mind. Joe said he could detect right away, by how a person used their body, whether they had sex recently and how much they liked it. That was surely a scary thought—realizing what Joe knew about me and many others. He allowed that sex, being the basis of existence, released something into your body that relaxed the muscles and deeply rested you in preparation for more sex. He was absolutely convinced that he could tell right away whether a person had a satisfactory sex life, particularly if that person was a woman. He talked about sex the same way he talked about exercise, but in this case, sex became a colleague of Contrology. I tried to imagine Joe having sex with a variety of his clients, some of whom I certainly fantasized about, but the picture never came into my head.

Strolling down the avenue, or, more precisely, charging down the avenue with Joe, was not only exercise, not only a seminar on how to walk and stand, not only an education in Contrology, but an insight into the mind of a man who had his hands on some of the most beautiful women's bodies in the world. I never saw even the slightest flash of anything sexual or improper about how he handled or treated anyone. He was focused on his work. What he did after work, or had done over the years, I had no idea. Joe for me back in the 1960s was certainly a breath of fresh air. And terribly liberating. Slowly the chains of a "proper" upbringing were loosening. And more rapidly my connections to Joe and Pilates were tightening. I sensed Joe could see both in my body.

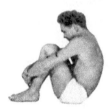

CHAPTER 4

A Far-Fetched Prophecy

Early on the morning of October 6, 1967, Clara called and told me Joe was in the emergency ward at Lenox Hill Hospital. She asked me to come over as soon as I could. "Joe and I need you."

"Sure," I said. "I will be there in about fifteen minutes."

I needed to get going, but she continued—unusual for her, as she and Joe were never comfortable on the phone, and even less so when she was at a nurses' station in a hospital. "This place is a madhouse and Joe is extremely difficult, although they have calmed him down with drugs. I think he will be okay." I didn't ask any questions.

I got the call because I had during the last few years become almost like family, and Clara didn't know who else to call. She needed help and could rely on me, a lifelong New Yorker. If Clara was the sick one instead of Joe, Joe, I am sure, would not call anyone, possibly not even 911. And if he did call 911, they would have had to sedate Joe even though he was not the patient, just to get Clara to the hospital. Joe hated doctors, hated medicine, and while everyone hates hospitals, he hated them more.

When I finally found the narrow room, more like a horse stall, where Joseph Pilates had been taken by ambulance less than an hour before, I saw Clara compressed into a corner behind the curtain that shielded Joe from the commotion in the hall. She had made herself barely visible. A sea of people in white hovered over Joe, and they talked to each other across his body as if he was not there . . . which in a certain way he wasn't. Those attending him who wore starched white caps (all women), the nurses, busied themselves with adjusting the plastic plumbing, placing monitoring sensors, and injecting medicine into the IV lines. Those without hats and with stethoscopes hanging from their necks (all men) were checking Joe physically and calmly giving instructions to the nurses in low, cryptic voices. The doctors and nurses on both sides of the bed were completely occupied with needles, tubes, masks, cuffs, bags of fluid. Heads nodded; notes were taken on clipboards. The pace was hurried, but not frantic.

Once I saw Joe's face through the screen of medical people, he didn't look too bad for an eighty-four-year-old man lying flat in a hospital bed. He had good color, despite harsh fluorescent lighting. His eyes were open. But there was no question this was a sick man. His arms were strapped to the bed, allowing some movement, but noticeably not enough to allow him to remove any of the plumbing feeding his body. His legs were similarly strapped down. He had oxygen tubes hooked around his ears and stuck into his nostrils. They were taped in place at his temples. His hair was a mess. His good eye, always hard to watch, moved around furtively as if he were trying to find out what was going on but couldn't.

Clara grabbed my hand as I poked my head around the curtain, and she pulled me to the foot of the bed, so Joe could see me.

A very muffled "Hello, John" came out in a quiet voice with Joe's permanent German accent. That murmur was about all Joseph Hubertus Pilates could muster.

Clara could fit into almost any space, but there was no room for me with all the personnel there. After a brief look in at Joe, we had to step out. Clara and I paced back and forth outside the room, in our states of shock, while the doctors and nurses did their work. This simply could not be happening! Joseph Pilates, the world's most fit octogenarian, helpless. Yesterday he taught Contrology all day; today he was flat on his back in an emergency room, breathing bottled oxygen.

"For the first time in forty years, Joe couldn't get out of bed this morning," Clara told me, quite calmly. "He complained that he couldn't get enough air in his lungs but insisted that if he lay back and cleared his lungs with deep exhales, using the springs and stuff attached to his V-Bed to help his body force the air out, he would be fine."

Clara went on: "He tried to grab something behind him, a wood bar attached to the bed with long springs, but he couldn't get it in front of him. He was so weak. He was gasping and gulping air as if drowning."

Clara told me that the minute Joe fell asleep, she called 911. He got crazy when she tried to call before. When they came, they forced an oxygen mask on his face. Joe was very weak. Even after they revived him with oxygen, he fell back when he tried to get out of bed.

Clara continued: "They restrained him and got a needle into his arm. Then they tied him down on a gurney and wheeled him into the elevator and then the ambulance. Joe yelled and protested all the way down the elevator, out onto Eighth Avenue, and into the ambulance. I followed. Joe was yelling so loudly, windows opened in the apartments facing the street. Then the ambulance left, and one of the men told me to take a cab to Lenox Hill Hospital."

I told Clara that I thought it was a very good hospital and happened to be where I was born.

***

As Clara finished filling me in, the nurses and doctors emerged from Joe's room in single file. They had to get on to the next emergency. One doctor dropped off from the white-robed swarm and talked to Clara and me in the hall. The doctor was young, very earnest, and clean-cut. He spoke in a flat tone and cadence, which was probably how he was trained to handle the chaos of his work and the anxiety of family members. He remarked that the patient (he didn't know the name) was resting comfortably and stabilized.

That was far from enough for me. "What is the cause of all this?"

The doctor said Joe had chronic compromised pulmonary function and now had pneumonia.

"Doctor, what is the prognosis?" I pressed on, thinking the use of a quasi-medical term might loosen him up. It didn't.

He looked down and away from Clara and me and said: "We are giving him antibiotics intravenously, keeping his fluid levels high, giving him oxygen, trying to keep him calm—not in his case an easy task—and watching all his vital signs, which are at the moment stable and satisfactory."

He looked up, as if embarrassed. His face softened. He remarked that Joe would not be sent to the critical care unit and would be admitted as a "pulmonary patient."

I inquired about the diagnosis.

The doctor said, "Pneumonia, complicated by emphysema. His lungs are scarred." He looked straight at me. "The patient is a tough man, and a fighter, always a good sign." I had my doubts. Clara thanked him.

Looking back, it is painfully obvious that given Joe's age and the cumulative threat of his deadly combination of lung diseases, the doctors had to know he was on the way out. Yet no one asked about family or suggested we should contact anyone. Maybe that had been handled with Clara on intake. I wonder if ER doctors ever get comfortable delivering bad news. As a lawyer, I never did.

I stayed a while, mostly for Clara, for whom they'd found a folding chair. Even though it was midmorning, I felt weak in the legs, so I leaned against the wall outside Joe's temporary room. Clara was okay and calm one minute, then suddenly jittery and barely coherent the next, probably from the fatigue of getting Joe to a hospital. Joe slept. I had a meeting at my office and had to leave the hospital, feeling guilty, sad, and worried. Clara planned to stay all day, and I hoped she could get some rest when Joe was settled in a private room. I told her I would check back later.

Around six o'clock in the evening, I left my office and took the Lexington Avenue subway back to the hospital. I was told at the reception desk where Joe was and found my way to his room. Clara had left a little while earlier. Joe couldn't look up as I entered. Now thoroughly oxygenated, hydrated, and undoubtedly sedated, he radiated ruddy good health, his white hair abundant but disheveled, his good eye bright and penetratingly blue.

I could see Joe concentrating on expanding his chest. He was straining under the neatly folded sheet. Joe had a weird bone in the middle of his chest that he could pop out at will, like the safety nipple on a pressure cooker. He was proud of that trick, which he did to show prospective clients his remarkable muscle control. I was certainly impressed when he first did it for me. But now he wasn't popping it out; some other pressure was.

Years later, I learned that the protruding bone was the result of rickets—a condition called "rachitic rosary." Childhood rickets—a vitamin D deficiency affecting calcification of the bones—was common in city kids at the time of Joe's youth. Joe had other hallmarks of the condition, too—his bowed or bandy legs, for example, and his oversized head. Joe never mentioned rickets and may have been unaware that he ever had it. He claimed dubiously that he began to develop his exercise program at an early age because he had asthma, which he overcame.

Despite breathing difficulties, with his good color there seemed to be some life in Joe, but only if you looked past the plastic tubing, connectors, valves, and needles in his arms and wrists; the plastic bags with fluid hanging from several posts and dripping medication into his veins; and the oxygen cannula in his nostrils taped to his face. His arms were still in restraints.

I sat in the stiff chair to the side of his bed and put my hand on top of his. He glanced sideways as if to see if I was friend or foe. He nodded and kept his hand under mine.

I asked if he would like me to read to him.

"You know some German?"

When I shook my head and said no, he told me not to bother.

"What about TV?"

"Never," he said.

We sat there in silence. He was too sedated, or too tired, or too weak to talk, and he was not very interested in listening to anything I had to say. He didn't care about the World Series or any other sport I could think of. The protests of American involvement in the Vietnam War were big news, but he was disinterested in the protests and the politics behind them. President Lyndon Johnson had just recently committed political suicide in a closely watched speech by escalating the United States involvement in the Vietnam War. Joe was unaware of the speech and the controversy, maybe even the war. Over the years with Joe I never found a topic for conversation unrelated to Contrology. Long silences were common and okay. He wasn't hostile or rude: he simply didn't want to talk or listen.

Despite the silence, I had a sense it was important to be in the room. Joe needed company; Clara needed to know she could leave. So I visited him daily, usually once early in the morning and then later in the evening. He wasn't improving, and this, plus the silence, made the visits gloomy and uncomfortable. I was just there—neither entertainment nor diversion. Whether my presence meant anything to Joe, I'll never know. I know it meant something to me.

During my visits, I would sit there gazing at the equipment and listening to the beeps, chirps, buzzes, and sounds coming from the technology monitoring Joe. I watched, for my own diversion, the colorful and dynamic graphs of his vital signs, oxygen, heartbeat, and blood pressure. Joe was suddenly a measurable object. On my second or third visit, the oxygen cannula in his nose was gone, and in its place, a clear plastic tent was over the top of the bed, held up by shiny steel tent poles. Not only was the tent ominous, it isolated Joe and hindered the little possibility of communication between us. The tent was by far the most disturbing piece of gear in the room, but after a while I got used to it. After an hour or so of hand-holding, Joe dozed off into a real sleep, so I left.

I stopped in for a visit Sunday morning, October 8, hoping to have a word or two with Joe and perhaps with someone on the staff who could give me some information. Sunday meant little medical staff and many family visits with lots of well-dressed people roaming the halls, carrying bright flowers and an occasional box of contraband chocolate. Only the nurse was around for my questions. She evaded all my attempts to get an indication of what lay ahead. The nurse was well practiced and good at sidestepping with the mantra "You will have to speak to the doctor." I wasn't family, and she wasn't allowed to say more. Joe seemed little different from the day before, certainly no worse.

When I returned to the hospital that evening, I could sense a difference from the morning. Clara had just left for the day. Joe was in the usual position beneath the oxygen tent, completely wired up; the gear in the room looked to be the same, but there was a different feel, almost a different smell. Joe was fading.

I sat down next to the bed in a plastic chair, at a forty-five-degree angle to the man I had studied with, walked with, eaten with, and listened to for the past four years. I slipped my hand under the edge of the oxygen tent and put it on top of Joe's. He was asleep. When I had stopped in earlier that morning, he had seemed more animated and a bit fidgety. That evening the nurse was in the room when I arrived, and she told me Joe had refused food for the first time that day. She also told me the attending physician was not ready to feed him intravenously.

Joe seemed paler than he had been that morning, and his breathing, while regular, was shallower and slower; I thought I detected a bit of desperation on the inhale. When he awoke, he twisted his head to see me, recognized me, grunted something, and turned back to facing up. His eyes were closed, and I fully expected he would doze off. But he didn't. He started to talk as if to an unseen audience even though I was right there. He seemed too tired, or sedated, or weak to have energy to talk, but that didn't stop him.

I couldn't tell if he was addressing the conversation to me, or just to anyone. Or even no one. When he inhaled, which was laborious, he couldn't speak, and when he spoke, he was short of breath. The words came out with difficulty in an unusually subdued voice with a scary vibrato. Once he got the words out, in bursts after each gulp of air, he was clear and distinct. I listened. I hoped he felt my hand and knew that I was there. I was concerned about the effort and energy he summoned to talk, but there was no way of stopping him. My sense was that there was a force within him compelling him to talk, to express and cleanse himself of some inner vexation.

His topic, as always: Contrology. This time, he talked about why it hadn't caught on. According to him, it was "just a matter of time—Contrology was perfect, people will awaken to their need of it to survive in the modern world. I was forty years too soon. The world will catch up." As always, optimism. He believed it. A sweet thought.

I sat there facing him, trying my best to let him know through exaggerated nods that I heard him and that I agreed—even though I didn't. Now and then I patted his hand. It took a lot of his precious energy to get all this off his chest, but with Joe Pilates, there was no way to head him off or divert him. I had never heard the "forty years too soon" rationale for the inability of Contrology to catch on. I could not imagine Contrology could or would continue without Joe. It was hardly surviving even with his dominating, evangelistic presence. But as I write this today, it turns out Joe's prediction was accurate. Tens of millions of people do Pilates.

Joe continued his ramble. What came out seemed driven by anger, perhaps disappointment at the failure of man's salvation to catch on. I had never accepted that Contrology was the ultimate cure-all. I had always listened attentively and not once was tempted to argue with Joe. I was afraid to dispute what he said, since it was not just questioning his statement, but really questioning his whole raison d'être: like questioning religious faith in the devout. This certainly was not the time to do so.

I had never had the courage to question Joe about his expectation that the world was supposed to adopt Contrology when only a few people knew about it. And I had an enduring question about the roots of Joe's faith. Did he need to be appreciated as a savior? Was this commercial propaganda? Was he seeking celebrity? Or, as I thought and still do, did he care about people's health? Perhaps, deep down, after his difficult and tumultuous life, he needed validation: validation from the medical profession. He wanted the profession to say his "cure" for the world's illnesses was effective and, as its creator, he merited great respect. He loved being needed and being respected. He most certainly would have adored it had his program obtained mass acceptance. Even without acceptance, professional endorsement supporting his work may have been enough.

Had I not been his enthusiastic student, and had I not heard this before, and had I not already come to grips with the pop-up lectures of Joe Pilates as the product of an obsessed and very passionate man, I would have thought he had slipped into some delusional phase. He said, and sincerely seemed to believe, "Doctors reject my system because they know it will work and then they will be out of business. No sickness, no patients, no money." The profession's indifference to him was, I believe, his most painful rebuke.

"Joe, maybe it's also because they like to play hero," I said. "Relax, stop talking, and save your strength."

But like the Energizer Bunny, he just kept going. Joe talked to the ceiling of his oxygen tent. He spoke about the several letters he wrote to the surgeon general of the United States, with whom he had a contact through a client. He promised he could help President Eisenhower fully recover from his heart attack. He couldn't believe his letters went unanswered. Joe talked about trying to present his system to the orthopedic societies in New York. He was never invited to make a presentation, which infuriated him. He told me he begged ballet dancers whom he had fixed to tell their ballet company doctors about his methods and gain an audience for him. Nothing came of that. He insisted, like a Baptist preacher, if everyone did Contrology, there would be no disease, no stress, and no war. Mankind, according to Joe, had a whole new enemy: the stress of the modern world. Doctors couldn't fix that; he could. Joe's anger was still there as he pushed words out, a good sign, even if muted by his breathing difficulties and muffled by the oxygen tent.

This was not the first time in the four years I had known him, worked with him, walked with him, ate with him, that I heard this anti-doctor lecture. But this time it came out differently, as if being read from a balky teleprompter. He spoke about how Contrology improved eating, sleeping, bathing, work, sex, and playing sports, and medicine didn't. Not that Joe's exercises had cured me of all emotional and physical ills, but they had certainly improved my life and physique. And something important had rubbed off from my contact with him inside and outside his gym. I had a different and far better attitude.

He continued to waste his precious energy talking. I knew I couldn't stop him, and then I thought by getting his story of frustration off his chest he might rest. On he went, doubling back and re-blasting the medical profession, "a bunch of greedy blockheads seeking only to keep people ill." Where he found the air or the strength to get all of this out, I couldn't imagine.

From moment to moment he jerked against the restraints as if he needed to use his hands and arms to express himself. Normally, Joe let his arms dangle when speaking, picking them up only for emphasis, almost like a boxer taunting his opponent and then using little punches as punctuation—jab for comma, uppercut for period, and both hands for exclamation point. He rested for a few minutes.

I had a moment to consider what he had said. Just as I finished reminding myself to continue my role as student at the foot of the master, Joe started up again, like a mobile phone whose battery wore down during a call and then got plugged into the wall. New subject this time: his current condition. He found renewed energy for this topic.

I remember him saying: "One month of exercises and I will be back. I need to force the blocked air out, so my lungs can work again. My exercises are perfect for this. Clean out dirty New York air, let in fresh New York air." As if New York air, particularly in his apartment and gym right above a bus stop, could ever be described as "fresh."

As Joe spoke, I imagined I was in the gym, with Joe leaning over me. I saw myself doing many of Joe's exercises, which sought to expand the chest through gaining flexibility in the rib cage and control over the diaphragm. I heard him commanding me to "breeze the air out, all out." He loved the exhale. It was the downbeat of his life's music. But Clara had obviously not told him about the pneumonia nor scar tissue from emphysema, neither of which could be turned around by exercise.

My little mental picture brought tears to my eyes from the pain of seeing him lie there, so helpless, so beaten by a force he couldn't combat. So often he had said: "I have never been sick for even a day in my whole life." His powerlessness against disease didn't square with his claims for Contrology, and I could tell he knew it.

Joe in a hospital was a rebuke to Contrology. But he had a defense. He once again blamed his lung condition on the "burning" of his lungs a few years before, when a fire broke out in his building. He had told me the story several times over the last four years. It came up, as it did now, whenever he breathed with difficulty or wheezed.

Around 1962, shortly before my time with him, a hot plate or bad wiring had started a fire in a rear apartment or the storeroom on Joe and Clara's floor. Smoke poured out of the front of the building. Joe told the story, nearly word for word the same every time, like this:

"The firemen came up the exterior fire escape on the Eighth Avenue side, forced open the windows to my gym, and rushed in. When they saw all my wood equipment, much of it in their way to the back of the building, they started to throw it out into the street even though there was no fire near it. They were throwing my life, my work, right out the window where it was kaput. So, I grabbed a pole and started swinging at them to stay away from my machines. They saw I meant it, and to clear the way they would have to throw me out too. One or two of them said okay and helped me pile the equipment up out of the way. I stayed there and guarded it. There was plenty of smelly, thick smoke, and I didn't have a mask like they did."

So typical of Joe—ready to fight, ready to challenge even burly, well-equipped New York City firemen, ready to look out for himself and take the world on single-handedly. Joe had inhaled a great deal of acrid smoke. His story was that he refused to go to the hospital, but others reported that he coughed so badly they took him by ambulance to Roosevelt Hospital around the corner. He left shortly after he got there, with or without permission. Maybe the ER happily let him go because they couldn't control him. He knew he had damaged his lungs. Nonetheless, he smoked the occasional cigar in his pipe.

Whatever Joe knew about emphysema or scar tissue on the lungs, he certainly did not believe they were permanent conditions. Not so long before this emergency, Joe told me he had fixed his lungs. He may have had a special connection with the human body, and particularly his, but he was no X-ray machine. He couldn't see into his lungs nor was he one to be honest with himself about how he felt. I admired his optimism and kept my doubts to myself.

His talk finally trailed off. He wore himself out and started to drift into sleep. But then he shook himself awake and whispered: "One day everyone in the world will know about Contrology and do it, and we won't need doctors, or hospitals." With that said, he dozed off. I left soon after. I, too, was tired, and I was sad and so jammed with emotion I was mentally numb.

I was the last nonmedical person to see Joe alive. His prediction may have been his last words. So unrealistic, I thought, but so good to die to.

And, as it would turn out, so accurate.

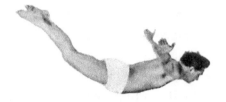

CHAPTER 5

Fortunately, He Had Disciples

The end came for Joseph Hubertus Pilates sometime early Monday morning, October 9, 1967, after a hard life. What was left of everything he learned about the structure and movement of the human body and how to exercise it was lodged with Clara, several dedicated assistants, a few teachers whom he had trained, and a group of maybe fifty regular clients, including my parents and me. There were photographs, home movies, and a book, but the maestro, the only one who understood it all, the only one who could transform what he knew of human movement into a program of exercise, was Joe. Or so we thought.

Joe died alone with his dreams unfulfilled, his discovery unappreciated, his business barely alive. Only Clara and I, and perhaps a few others, had been with him during his last few days while he lay nearly unconscious in a hospital bed. He had neither fame, nor money, nor descendants. Yet right before he took his last labored breath, he was optimistic because of his faith in his exercise program. Today his name is known throughout the world, heard on television, in movies and novels and magazines, even on Broadway. His dream has been fulfilled; his discovery loved and practiced everywhere, the focus of hundreds of how-to books, DVDs, and monographs, and the basis for businesses in almost every country.

That Monday afternoon I helped Clara close the gym and make the arrangements for Joe's funeral. Clara knew Joe was a Mason, so we called them, and they took over the preparations. I taped a handwritten sign on the gym door saying that Joe had died, and that the gym would be closed for a week. I didn't call the assistants or the clients. Clara had the numbers, and she said she would call the senior assistant, John Winters, and he would call the others. We put an obituary in all the New York papers—and there were a handful of papers back then. I received calls asking about the services, and I provided the details or the phone number of the Masonic lodge where Joe was a member.

Shortly after Joe's funeral in 1967, Clara asked me to help her take care of his affairs and get them in order. She arrived at my office a few days later, dressed not in her nurse's outfit but in her "going out" clothes. The same outfit she wore at Joe's funeral. I was always a little surprised to see Clara not in her nurse's clothes. It was a rare occasion. Coming to a midtown law firm, at least for her, was akin to a state visit: proper dress obligatory. There she was in her finery: a dark skirt and blouse, a necklace, a small hat with attached fake veil perched at a rakish angle on her gray, short, perfectly combed hair, and sensible brown leather lace-up shoes. She had walked and bused across town and then downtown.

Despite the radical change of outfit, the lady in my office was still Clara: the frail, nurse-like person whom I first saw standing behind Joe in the gym, several years earlier. She was carrying a Bloomingdale's shopping bag (I never forgot that—Bloomingdale's being so unlike Clara!) along with her small gray leather purse, like the one Queen Elizabeth carried. There wasn't any indication on her face or in her manner that her husband had just died. She and Joe were masters at hiding emotion. I could tell from her voice she was sad and very frightened, but this was business, and emotions could not get in the way. I, too, had to rein mine in.

Clara laid out the contents of her shopping bag on my conference table. They consisted of a small handgun—a loaded German Walther PPK 7.65 mm (secret agent 007's preferred concealed-carry weapon), a box of ammunition, an envelope containing $1,000 in cash, and two or three letters to Joe inquiring about licensing Contrology. That was it. I was taken aback but guessed Clara had no idea what was involved in settling an estate and just hadn't brought the necessary papers. I took out a pad and started to make a list as I told her what I required. I first asked about their tax returns. Clara said there were none. I asked why not. She said Joe never did a tax return. They had been in the United States forty-one years and never filed a federal, state, or city tax return? I asked if there had been any trouble, any inquiries?

Her answer: "No."

I moved on. "Did Joe have a social security number?"

Her answer: "I don't know."

At this point, I suspected the answer to a lot more questions but still had to push on. I lifted the pen from the pad, thinking I didn't need to have a list of my client's crimes.

"What about your marriage license?"

"We never got officially married."

This was getting heavy.

"Any bank accounts?"

"No."

"Where did you put the money from the business?"

"We hid it."

"What about checks?"

"Didn't take them or credit cards, only cash."

"So I take it you paid for everything in cash?"

"Yes."

"And you paid the assistants in cash?"

"Yes."

"What about workmen's compensation insurance?"

"What is that?"

"Do you have a lease for your apartment or the gym?"

"Years ago, I think. I don't have any papers."

"The house in New Hampshire—who owns it?"

"A friend."

Finally, one last question: "Clara, did Joe ever become a US citizen?"

This was a test. And she passed. She knew he had and said so. They both had US passports, although I never saw Joe's. There was no sense going any further down this path.

What Clara wanted from me, what she desperately needed but couldn't ask for, even if she'd been conscious of it, had nothing to do with the estate. If there were assets, she was not telling me about them. It had everything to do with what was to happen to the business—and to her. The unthinkable, the unimaginable, had happened: Joe Pilates was gone, and she was still here. She had no family, no money. She had an iron will and clients of the gym who loved her. Looking back, Clara desperately needed help and didn't need anyone peeking into Joe's past.

I excused myself to go to the men's room for a few minutes, so I could think about what I had just heard. Could this indifference to civil requirements continue? What were the consequences for Clara? What if Joe's obituary or death certificate triggered an investigation into the couple's business and they came after her? No one could uncover Joe's background or his affairs because there were no records, according to Clara. He immigrated and became a citizen. Those were public records. Tax records were private.

When I did the usual lawyer's risk analysis, I concluded that anything bad coming from Joe's conduct was unlikely. The chances of discovery slight, the consequences insignificant. Joe, I thought, had gotten away with it. Even if some official investigated and discovered that Joe defaulted on his legal obligations and assessed significant liabilities and penalties for failure to file and pay, what could they do to Clara? She wasn't even his wife. Attach her nonexistent bank account? And she could claim truthfully that Joe ran everything. Since the estate had no assets (at least any I knew about), there was no need to transfer anything from Joe's name to Clara's. There was absolutely nothing for me to do—except deal with the illegal pistol in my possession.

The pistol, a German Luger or, as we called it around the office, the "Bob Seed Special," I put in the office safe. Although it was illegal to possess a firearm in New York City without a near-impossible-to-get permit—which Joe didn't have—I wasn't too concerned.

The pistol had an interesting legal story because of its use as an effective alternative to a covenant not to compete. One morning, while Joe was still alive, I had arrived at an empty gym. Bob Seed, Joe's early morning assistant, wasn't there. Joe burst in and asked me if Bob Seed had contacted me.

I said he hadn't and asked why. Joe told me Bob had opened a gym across town and was contacting and stealing Joe's clients, particularly the early morning ones like me. I offered my help and suggested I write a letter. Joe said: "Never mind, I'll take care of it. Are you okay by yourself this morning?"

I said, "Sure." And Joe left. About one-half hour later, Joe returned and said, "I took care of it."

I asked, "What did you do?"

"I went to Seed's new gym, took my gun out from behind me, put it up to his forehead, and said, 'Call one more of my clients and I'll be back and pull the trigger.'"

The gun was Joe's version of a non-compete provision in a legal document. It was certainly quicker, cheaper, and more effective than any legal instrument I could have prepared, or anything I could have said to convince Bob Seed not to steal any of Joe's clients. That what Joe did constituted multiple felonies did not seem to cross his mind, much less inhibit him.

The sight of Joe striding across Manhattan in his gym shorts with a deadly, unlicensed pistol sticking out was not comforting. Joe, like most everyone else, knew the gun laws in New York, and he must have known that he had no legal remedy against Seed. There was no employment agreement, no non-compete clause, absolutely nothing to prevent Seed from contacting Joe's customers. Except Joe's remedy:

his trusty German-made Walther PPK. It worked. Clara didn't want the pistol so she brought it to my office, thinking I could get rid of it. Within months, Lady Luck looked down upon my Good Samaritan act, accepting a hot pistol, and the mayor decreed a one-month amnesty for turning in illegal firearms, no questions asked. I will never forget the detective's eyes when he saw this German-made gem of a gun. He apologized about not being able to give me a receipt ("This has to be kept anonymous . . .") as he slipped the gun into his jacket pocket.

**

I still wonder why I wasn't curious when Clara told me about Joe's astonishing disregard for the ordinary requirements of every citizen. One reason is that criminal defense lawyers rarely ask their clients the simple question: "Did you do it?" In the almost ten years I had been out of law school, many weird situations had crossed my desk. It was not unusual to have clients who failed to file a tax return or two. Easily remedied. It was not unusual, although back then rare, to have unmarried clients living as a married couple for a long time. There was social pressure to get married (which Joe and Clara avoided by telling everyone they were) and tax reasons to get married (which didn't apply to them since they paid no taxes). But no social security number, no bank account, no driver's license—these violations were novel. The situation before me was as bizarre as it was mysterious. I just let it slide on by. My concerns at the time were focused on Clara's survival and the continuation of the gym, which were tightly linked. Could the cadre of Contrology enthusiasts, of which I was one, keep the gym operational and support Clara? Could either be done without Joe?

For quite some time after Joe's death, questions niggled into my head about his behavior. Why had Joseph Pilates so carefully avoided all contact with the government? He made himself invisible to the government, yet he was in a world where he was a visible person and he certainly enjoyed acclaim. There had to be a reason. Joe knew about rules, regulations, paperwork, and all that. He had escaped Germany, avoided military service, immigrated to the United States, and applied for and become a citizen, and yet he intentionally avoided any other contact with the government. Joe was either a naughty boy harboring a problem with authority and/or distrust of government, or he had done something in the past that he needed to keep hidden. I had to admire his chutzpah, but his behavior raised a few questions. If he had been hiding something, what was it and why had it ruled his life?

After the Clara revelations, for about a year, I had these little moments of anxiety about Joe's house of cards falling in. I just air-brushed away the thought that something was amiss. Even if I had wanted to dig, where to start? With Clara? It was doubtful she would reveal very much, even if she knew. Joe and Clara had been at this for a long time. Not until I began this book, when I tried to unravel the Pilates story and had to put things in order, did the questions I had so easily brushed off become hard to ignore.

That day when Clara came to see me at my office, I assured her I would take care of what she needed, and I returned the envelope with the cash; I told her that she needed so little there would be no charge. Clara thanked me for helping her and fought me, unsuccessfully, for a few moments on the $1,000. After shaking my hand, she put on her well-worn coat, and we walked together toward the elevator. At that point, neither of us knew what would be involved going forward. Clara's predicament was the first concern. The only solution was keeping Joe's gym operating.

So here I was in 1967, trying to earn my keep as a junior partner in a medium-sized law firm. From worrying about obtaining, servicing, and billing clients, with a few weekly breaks to get to Joe's gym and to play squash, I was now additionally worried about Clara Pilates and keeping Joe's gym going. Up to then I had avoided being in "business." My dad was in business and he didn't seem to like it, escaping as frequently as he could to play cards in the afternoon with his friends. I wasn't even interested in the business of my new law firm. I was there to bring in clients and litigate. My partners took care of the books, and the profit and loss statement, cash flow, and borrowing from the bank. Now suddenly I had a very sketchy exercise business on my shoulders. I didn't ask for it, seek it, or know what to do with it. But I got it.

Joe's gym and Joe's Contrology were stumbling toward extinction. Both had been all Joe and just Joe. Joe's gym hadn't been a viable business for quite some time. It must have been enough to sustain him and Clara, or they had enough cash hidden away to make ends meet. But it had to be on the cusp of actual bankruptcy. Joe's Contrology was randomly documented mostly in photographs on his wall. A few of his assistants and students knew Contrology perfectly. I doubt they had any idea about the financial health of the business. Except perhaps if Joe couldn't meet payroll.

Clara and I decided to reopen a week later. We put a note on the door, she called the assistants, and we all made calls. Everyone returned. It was as if Joe were still alive. The clients continued to come and do their workouts. Joe's assistants maintained their schedules and took excellent care of the clients exactly as if Joe were in the room supervising. Clara was ever present. Joe had trained everyone well— the gym seemed to run itself. Strange that everything seemed to function with Joe gone.

I even expected Joe to show up. That the gym continued to operate is testimony to Joe's belief that Contrology was something fundamental to human existence. There was something deeper about Contrology that gave it life independently of its creator. Many years later, I saw the irony behind it all: Joe had managed the business side so minimally—Contrology being to him *much* more than a science or a commercial venture; to him it was an art and a study—that his absence as a manager had no effect. Anyone could collect five dollars at the door and give it to Clara. There were no records, no appointments to be made, no releases or waivers or consents, no forms to file, no insurance claims, not even towels. Someone (maybe Clara) came in to clean up at the day's end. Once a week, someone oiled the machines. Joe's assistants put everything back in place before they left every evening. Joe's gym was, it seemed, a perpetual motion machine.

Nevertheless, there had to be a boss, and Clara couldn't do it.

***

To help find a new manager, I contacted our cadre of loyal customers. One evening we had a meeting in the gym. About twenty people showed up. Seeing people sitting around on the exercise equipment, fully dressed and talking, would have driven Joe up the wall. The attendees resolved to keep the gym operating and to take care of Clara. Julie Clayburgh, Arthur Steel (my father), and I were nominated (not by us) to be the "executive committee" and we were unanimously confirmed. No one wanted the unwinnable responsibility of keeping the gym running, yet no one wanted their attachment to Contrology to be finished.

None of the three of us knew how to run the gym, which had been limping along the last few years even before Joe died. Without the maestro, there seemed to be no possibility that it could continue much longer, any more than LaGuardia Airport could operate without a control tower. None of us knew how much money Joe and Clara made or how much the assistants were paid. I suspected the landlord was the only person with a steady income from the gym, and even that was questionable.

A few of us close to Clara were immediately concerned for her well-being. She was not all that strong and had very poor vision, and while she was an excellent backup for Joe, she was no substitute. She seemed to depend on Joe, and the gym, for her survival. Joe's assistants, like Clara, were there to help, but they, too, did not have any interest in managing a gym or possess what it takes to be the chief instructor: passionate about Contrology, sufficiently charismatic to attract and retain clients, empathetic, intuitive about everyone's body, and that *je ne sais quoi* teaching quality that inspires the student to dig deeper. Nor did they know how to deal with injuries or common aches and pains. Without someone with those skills and abilities, it wouldn't be long before the clientele would stop attending, the assistants would lose interest, and Clara would be left without a purpose in life and nothing to sustain her economically. That is what we thought, at least.

We were wrong.

The first surprise of course was that the clients and Joe's assistants continued as if nothing had happened. Also, as I mentioned, very little managing had to be done.

But the other big surprise was that many clients approached one of us to say they were prepared to do what they could to keep the gym going. Suddenly, we went from a group of people not allowed to talk to each other in the gym to a community. No one was going away.

The gym's instant rebound from Joe's death proved his point: Contrology was the main attraction, not Joe nor any individual. The Pilates of today is further proof that Joe's confidence in his program was well-placed. Whatever Joe imbedded into certain of his students not only stuck but, like roots blindly seeking water, kept us motivated to ensure its survival. We wanted the gym to be there for selfish reasons— we wanted to have a place so we could keep doing Contrology—but that was not only because we liked it. We, too, had caught the Joe bug and believed in the importance, almost the genius, of Contrology.

I discovered many years later that during two separate periods, in the 1940s and 1950s, Joe's clients had set up a not-for-profit company or a foundation to preserve Contrology and to provide for some continuity upon his death. That involved a lot of volunteer effort, a lot of organizing, and many meetings, all for the love of Contrology. The idea was to have an entity "own" Contrology to ensure its perpetuation. In exchange, Joe was to remain in charge of the gym, construct the archive, and assist in getting everything down on paper, and he and Clara would receive a guaranteed income for their lives.

Unfortunately, these efforts ended badly because of terrible conflicts between Joe and the members. The conflicts were all attributed to Joe's protectiveness and constant but unjustified fear that the members of the new organization were seeking to exploit or control his work and not to preserve it. Quite the opposite: Joe just wouldn't let go, even to people who were his students, who loved the work and had nothing to gain but the assurance that Contrology had a shot at perpetual existence. Joe just couldn't allow anyone, no matter how benevolent, to have control over his "baby." Was it because he thought others would have the power to "change" Contrology, or reinterpret it, or teach it improperly, or capitalize on it? Joe was trapped between, on the one hand, his aspiration that Contrology become a widely taught and universally practiced regimen, which required open access, and, on the other, his inability to let anyone near its "source code." If only he could see Pilates as the open system it is today!

While Joe was alive, I did not know about his break with those who wanted to help him perpetuate his discovery. After his death I found a document showing that my mother, Ruth, had been a member of the foundation that Joe rejected. She was even on the education committee. My mother had no memory of being a member of any foundation or having attended any meetings. Her dues of ten dollars per year, not evidenced by a check—probably paid in cash—did not indicate strong participation. Nor would she have tolerated and remained involved in any situation involving internal feuding and contentiousness, which was what inevitably occurred when Joe thought others might have a say in his activity.

On one of my many walks with Joe, he mentioned that people were always trying to steal his work, but he had stopped them. He gave me no specifics. It reminds me of the Apple Computer company in its early days, wanting everyone to buy its computers but not allowing anyone near the code for the operating system. It worked for Apple initially, but eventually Apple had to cave on some parts of its system just to compete. Joe's crazy protectiveness left Clara, and anyone else interested in Contrology's continuity, with nowhere to turn.

Joe didn't train anyone to take over after his time was up. Back in the 1960s, physical therapy was rarely chosen as a career. You couldn't make a living. There were very few athletic clubs for the public, certainly none of the large franchises of today. There were no customers. Teaching Contrology as a profession was unmarketable—no one had ever heard of it. Joe's successor had to first learn to do Contrology, then learn to teach it (a different skill), and had to be a missionary and salesperson to get others to do it. Looking back, Joe had been wrong to reject help. He had left us with no good options.

***

When we were conscripted as the executive committee, none of the three of us—my father, Julie Clayburgh, and I—expected we would have to actually run the gym. I'm not sure what we thought, if anything. But someone had to be in charge. And no one else stepped up, so we did it. We had one enormous advantage over those who had tried to help in the past: we did not have to deal with Joe.

The three of us just wanted to keep the gym operating for the use of our small community of aficionados, and to support Clara. We had no burning desire, probably never thought about it, to ensure the propagation, much less survival, of Contrology past our little confederation. We were not out to guard its purity or to turn a profit. We did what was required because no one else wanted to.

The first objective, keeping the doors open at 939 Eighth Avenue, the only place on the planet where the clientele could continue their well-settled routine, was not that difficult. Fortunately, there were a few longtime devoted assistants. When one of our gang of three managers called and said we would keep the Pilates's gym operating, whatever it took, the assistants were enormously relieved and prepared to work out a schedule and join the team to keep it going. Clara was still quite capable of paying (in cash) the rent and utilities, and very willing to come to the gym every day to lend her deep understanding of the work. Her presence was vital to the notion of continuity. And lastly, over the years the clientele had been winnowed down to a cadre of self-motivated individuals capable of taking care of themselves in the gym with a minimum of instructional assistance.

We were buying time and desperately needed Clara's presence to assure the clientele that Joe was still with them in a real way. The equipment had to be maintained—it was already long in the tooth—and fortunately Mr. Desio, who periodically came in to fix the equipment in the past, agreed to stop by more frequently. And one client, a busy businessman, volunteered to come in early every morning and make sure the equipment was properly oiled, cleaned, and ready for the stress of the day ahead.

Busying ourselves with the immediate problem allowed us to ignore the long-term issue of how to replace the person we thought to be irreplaceable. Who could fill Joe's shoes, attract and take care of new business, and inspire everyone to focus on the work and do their best? No one we could think of. Fortunately, the details of our daily efforts were enough to obscure this much bigger, unsolvable problem, so we limited our focus to the immediate tasks of staying open and making sure Clara was okay. We, like Joe, became minimalists and confined our attention to the moment and not the future.

The gym was a tired, old machine running down slowly, relying only on ancient momentum with no new energy. While our gang of three was injecting *some* new energy, and a bit of day-to-day working capital, our management team was makeshift and scattershot with no hope it could be sustained for long—so we thought. We operated day to day, hand to mouth, but we operated. Certainly an unconventional way to run a business, but then again, this was hardly a business. This was a club for us and a living for Clara.

I have no distinct memory of how the three of us worked together, which suggests it, too, was dictated by the doctrine of ease. We had no structure. We didn't hold meetings. There were lots of phone calls, and the gym just seemed to carry on. It got cleaned, the bills were paid, the cash receipts were accounted for, and our client base stayed pretty much the same. We were treading water; it is a wonder the business survived. Only if chaos is a business plan could anyone say we had one. But our fly-by-the-seat-of-our-pants approach worked to the extent that we kept the business alive—for two and a half years. That period of coasting finally brought us to a standstill—level ground. We could go no further. We had kept the small customer base together and involved. But we never had a long-range plan. Our objective after Joe's death was to keep the gym open and take care of Clara. That objective had run its course; it was time to get serious and be businesslike.

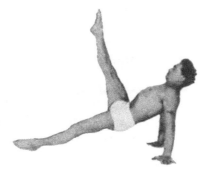

CHAPTER 6

We Heard the Fat Lady Singing

The inexperienced committee formed to perpetuate Contrology had, through miraculous nonmanagement, kept the doors open for two and one-half years after Joe's death, but barely. We, individually and as a committee, and the gym, had hit bottom. We were out of money, out of energy, without professional management. We were adrift with no land in sight. We had to do something. Our stopgap measures had run their course. We were at a crucial fork in the continuation of Contrology: close the doors or make it work.

In 1970 we assembled a larger group and started work on a long-term plan. Without a plan and everyone's support, we were done. We had dropped below the sustainability threshold. The larger group implored us to keep going and pledged involvement and money. And even then, we had to limp along for an indefinite period until we put together the pieces for a new, rejuvenated Pilates.

Our assets: Contrology and a cadre of regular and enthusiastic adherents. Among them were successful business people, prominent members of the dance and theater world, and a number of wealthy clients.

Arthur Steel, Julie Clayburgh, and I sent out a notice to every client, requesting their attendance at a meeting to discuss whether to close the doors or reorganize with a long-range plan, proper management, and working capital. And a plan to take care of Clara.

I prepared our introductory remarks, trying to boil down the pros and cons of our alternatives. On one side of the decision matrix, we had an existing not-for-profit business in the true sense of the expression, with several assets: a program of exercise, equipment, several experienced and loyal instructors, and a group of dedicated customers, some with money.

In the other column of the ledger, we had no marketing, no interest in our service, a moral and personal obligation to take care of Clara (Did Joe *anticipate* and *count upon* us to do this?), and no other way to continue to do our beloved Contrology.

To force us to decide, our landlord indicated he would not renew the lease because a well-funded dance company wanted our space. Even if we had a plan, no business model worked. After the rent was paid (and it would certainly go up), Clara was cared for and supported, and the assistants paid (sometimes from a payment received from a client minutes before or a quick loan from one of the three of us), there was nothing left. We had no working capital, no reserve, no line of credit. Just like before Joe's death. There was no reason to have any confidence we could attract more customers without Joe's star power, and there was a limit to the fee we could charge.

The meeting was in my law office, and I had to borrow extra chairs. Even then it was standing room only, everyone with long, sad faces. Among those present we had management, marketing, business-oriented people side by side with artists, writers, and Broadway composers and producers. Even in New York, this was a powerful group. Powerful and savvy, but somber; no one needed to be convinced that the gym was in a death spiral.

I chaired the meeting, and after struggling to get order, I was able to set the stage for a discussion of the simple question: "Where do we go from here—home or to a reborn, self-sustaining gym providing Contrology?" Once the floor was opened to comment, it was obvious: No one came to the meeting thinking it was a wake or to sit shiva for a deceased Pilates. They came to see if there was a way to keep it going because it meant so much to everyone.

Joe's Contrology, which we all agreed we would now call "Pilates," was a sustaining part of their lives. The attendees were prepared to do what they could to help. Among our group were several entrepreneurs: men and women who had started businesses from scratch and built them into profitable firms. They had seen worse turned into success. And they loved risk and challenge. They would participate with others in the room to provide capital for a fresh start to make the gym self-sustaining. We had what I mistakenly thought was the hard part—money. Looking back, the impetus to keep going was solely driven by everyone's addiction to Pilates—it had become a habit. No one mentioned the need to keep Joe's Contrology alive because one day millions would benefit from it. Our motivation was personal. And that was enough.

The enthusiasm to carry on had a downside for the three of us on the ad hoc executive committee, who wanted no further responsibility. Julie Clayburgh, Arthur Steel, and I had originally volunteered right after Joe's death two and one-half years earlier to be an interim management team. Now the group insisted we had to continue as the executive committee, not, I am sure, because we had done such a splendid job, but simply because no one was prepared to take our places. When the three of us jumped in initially, it was only to keep things going. Now we would have investors, a business plan, long-term goals. Our new role carried serious responsibilities. None of us were experienced. We weren't from the world of physical conditioning. We weren't dancers, athletes, physical therapists, wannabe teachers. We were just New Yorkers hooked on Pilates. And our management, such that it was, had led the gym slowly to the precipice of extinction. The group assured the three of us that the present dire circumstances were not our fault. Everyone in the assembled group understood there had been a complete lack of long-term planning, just like with Joe before his death, and just like with our management team. No one could fault us for losing the way simply because we never had a destination.

I asked who was to do the planning, who was going to do the actual work. My father was unavailable. Julie Clayburgh and I were busy with our own responsibilities. Someone suggested not to worry about anything but solving the day-to-day problems. When I pointed out that the day-to-day problems were everything necessary to reverse our predicament and that it required a real business plan in addition to capital, the room was silent.

I heard from someone, "Okay, you made your point. Now what can we do?" That broke the ice and launched a spirited discussion. The consensus was that the pledge of sufficient working capital was just a start. Everyone agreed that we needed a new, more centrally located and appealing space and a gifted manager-teacher. I pointed out that finding a well-located, affordable space for a noisy, trafficked gym was a challenge. And finding someone able to continue Joe's exercise routine, instill the benefits into others, and attract new clients while managing the operation seemed impossible.

Everyone agreed that a working group of about eight people from the attendees was necessary, and that the group had to commit to attend weekly meetings and take on a good bit of the legwork. When the meeting broke up, I was unsure about who was doing what, but I decided to wait until the first meeting of the working group to go into full panic mode. The thought crossed my mind that no task is too difficult for the person who does not have to do it. But the positive energy in the room, and hands raised when help was requested, quickly suppressed that bit of negativity.

The first step was to create a legal structure. We agreed that I should incorporate 939 Studio Corp. as a NY for-profit entity. Hope winning over experience. The working group began holding weekly meetings. We formed committees, assigned tasks, and developed a business plan. Everyone agreed to serve on one or more committees. I ran the weekly meetings, took notes, worked on a to-do list, served coffee, scheduled the next meeting, and suddenly realized this would be my continuing role.

From these meetings, a plan developed. We agreed that if Pilates was to survive in the world of the 1970s, it had to at least join and become part of the culture of the '70s. The facility had to have a modern, crisp appearance, and the vibe had to be high energy and fun. We needed a midtown New York address near where a large part of our customer base worked or shopped and close to dancers who brought great energy into the gym. But depending on dancers to support a business (other than Capezio and Philip Morris) was not realistic. Especially if the business was to be classy. One danger was becoming too classy, which would discourage dancers who loved a certain amount of grunge (it proved how dedicated they were). Clean grunge was acceptable. A style between chic, for the paying customers, and casual, for the dancers, both of whom were essential, had to be found.

We had several things going for us. Joe's assistants knew the work and had a deep commitment to it. They had kept it going without guidance after Joe's death. We had the gear—the Reformers, the Chairs, the Tower, the Guillotine, and the Ladder Barrel. We had Clara's full cooperation. She had no alternative. It was us or nobody. And, as a group, we had a good deal of worldly experience in fashion, business, the performing arts, and even construction and real estate. We were a bunch of smart, well-connected New Yorkers who knew how to get what we wanted. And we all wanted the same thing: to continue doing Pilates as if Joe were still with us.

With the objectives defined, a sense of enthusiasm developed among those volunteering to assist in bringing back Pilates from near-certain death. We could see, or thought we could see, a way out of the coma. People stepped up to take on various tasks. A relocation committee was formed. A business-plan committee sprang to life. A fundraising committee got together, and a "take care of Clara" group volunteered. Julie Clayburgh and I were assigned the task of finding Joe's replacement and, if that wasn't enough, took on the responsibility for the overall management of our shared enterprise. We were motivated. We felt it might work. It was exciting at the beginning, like a love affair. And perhaps as mindless.

Julie was a Broadway show producer. She was good at casting, at finding people—not only actors—to fill positions. Hopefully that would help in the search for Joe's replacement. The job description was daunting: run a gym on a shoestring where only Pilates was taught (no steam bath, no sauna, no makeup mirrors, no shaving cream), teach Pilates like Joe did, teach others to teach Pilates (like Joe didn't), supervise all the teachers and clients, get publicity to attract new business, deal with new clients, maintain Joe's standards, keep the equipment and the facility clean and running, and operate in the black. Where to look for such a person?

We knew we couldn't replace Joe or duplicate him. He was unique. He couldn't even do some of the things we sought in our new manager. The rubric that no one is indispensable kept running through our minds, although Joe seemed to be the exception that proved the rule. We didn't need a clone of Joe; we needed at least two of him. After all, people taught ballet and gymnastics, so we could find someone to teach Pilates. It wasn't that hard—we had all learned it.

Who, we wondered, knew Pilates well enough to teach it? We started with Joe's two primary assistants, Hannah Sakamirda and John Winters. Julie and I asked them what role, if any, they wanted to have in the "new, born again" Pilates. The answer: "The same as we have now and had under Joe—helping out." Neither wanted to manage; neither wanted to teach newcomers. Their loyalty was appreciated, their knowledge of Pilates essential, but our search had to continue.

The next panel of prospects included the few people already teaching outside the gym. These were Eve Gentry, Kathy Grant, Carola Trier, and Mary Bowen. Sadly, not one of them had the slightest interest. Eve Gentry, a gifted teacher with Joe's uncanny sensitivity to the workings of the human body, had relocated to Santa Fe and was well on her way to establishing a new outpost of Pilates. Kathy Grant, another outstanding teacher in Joe's mold, who had worked for Carola Trier and then become one of two people "certified" by Joe, was exceptionally busy training dancers and running a Pilates mini-studio in Henri Bendel—NY's very tony department store. There she could work with dancers for free while she took high fees (for those days) from Bendel's wealthy clientele. Carola Trier and Mary Bowen were very content with their mini-studios, and they didn't want the headache of a new clientele, the responsibility of attracting new customers, nor the administration of a new business.

We suggested to each prospective teacher we would find another person to take over the management side of the business, if they would take care of the teaching of Pilates. We begged, we played the guilt card ("We need you to continue Joe's work"), we promised a rose garden—anything, because we were desperate. The fanciest studio in the world was worthless without someone who could teach. But none of them bit.

With nowhere else to turn to find an experienced teacher, Julie and I finally decided we would have to settle on someone who knew and did Pilates and was willing to teach it, helped by the current assistants. I thought Clara might identify any former students who seemed to have an aptitude for Joe's program. After some thought, Clara suggested I contact Romana Kryzanowska, who Clara said studied with Joe enthusiastically some years earlier as a young, ambitious, but injured ballet dancer. Clara gave me the whole story. Soon after Joe fixed Romana (Joe was like an automobile mechanic working on "broken" dancers), she ran off to Peru with a wealthy, older Peruvian gentleman. Years and two children later, the marriage ended, and she returned to New York with her kids. Clara thought that Romana taught ballet somewhere in the city. Romana had stayed in touch with Joe over the years, was at Joe's funeral, and told Clara she still did Contrology. Joe had liked her. He thought she was a very good student. Clara suspected Joe may have had a brief affair with her. Romana was a gorgeous and very seductive nineteen-year-old at the time, and according to Clara, young dancers were hard to resist, particularly for someone in Joe's position with his (according to her) very active sex drive. Anyhow, Clara thought I should contact her and see if she was interested.

I located Romana and set up a meeting at a coffee shop on Columbus Avenue near her apartment. I was seated when Romana arrived with a typical high-energy flourish. She was forty-eight years old when we met in 1972. She didn't look like a ballerina. Even though short and stocky, she had that almost unmistakable relaxed, easy movement dancers favor when they are off duty. And a winning, somewhat wicked smile, flashing eyes, a great deal of almost wild hair, and a raspy, sexy voice. She dressed with an artsy flair, and it was easy to see that when younger she had been a very seductive creature. From her appearance and body language, I detected more than a little diva about her. Not a bad thing when looking for a Joe replacement. She was full of life and, just at first sight, seemed to be who we needed.

Romana, when she sat down, indicated that she had "heard" a group was trying to keep Joe's business alive, and she had a note from Clara saying I would call on her. Romana was several years older than I was. She was terribly suspicious of me. She started on the attack.

"Did you work for Joe? Are you working for Clara?" When I told her about our little committee, who they were, what they wanted to accomplish, and why I had sought her out, she listened but said nothing.

Then, after an uncomfortable silence, she told me she thought highly of Joe, whom she called "Uncle Joe," seemed to like but not love Clara, and deeply respected the work that she claimed to do every day.

Then the bomb: "I have no interest in managing a Contrology studio. I am a ballet teacher, have a son who is a rising star in the New York City Ballet, and am very happy with my life and don't need the thankless task of managing and teaching Contrology, thank you very much though." The real deal breaker was the part of the rather loose job description that required her to manage a studio and teach ordinary people, not dancers. She thought this job was beneath her. Ballet was her passion. Ordinary people were not Romana people—they were outsiders to the world of ballet, which was all that Romana cared about. My lack of ballet credentials (being an enthusiastic audience member was not enough) together with my suspicious involvement with Clara and Joe were insurmountable hurdles. We left with no later contact planned. I was more than a little stung by Romana's dismissive arrogance.

Obviously, I had failed. But despite the feeling I had been played with, worse, condescended to, there was something about Romana I thought could work. She could take over and run Pilates. She knew and loved movement, she could teach, she bristled with energy, and she was very commanding. Her ballet-world membership was an attraction. And I saw a little of Joe in her charisma and in her prima donna affect. I simply had no idea how to convince her. Whatever bait I had put on the hook was unattractive to her. It hadn't merited even a nibble.

I have attended many negotiations over the years of my law practice, and I have watched master negotiators at work. Acting indifferent to a proposal is a fundamental strategy. The trick for the other negotiator is to figure out whether the indifference is sincere or a tactic. If it is sincere, as I concluded about Romana's indifference, then the failure of any proposal was insurmountable. Romana was not negotiating for better terms, I was sure. She was being polite and listening to something that didn't appeal to her.

I reported back to Clara, who was not at all surprised. She said that most ballet people are very conservative and, except for what they do onstage, are exceptionally careful and afraid of taking chances. "Don't take it personally, John, ballet dancers tend to see themselves as different, better in fact, than everyone else. They did that to Joe and me from time to time. Joe paid no attention, but I was bothered."

Clara thought Romana might be different. Romana had kids, was divorced, suffered from unfulfilled high aspirations, and was well past her performance years. Then she said: "Try again, John, but do something differently."

I asked what. Clara said: "Try to think of something she would like, something arty, not something like work. Dancers work hard but don't understand work as we do." And she added, if Romana saw me again, it would mean there was a possibility. Clara, like Joe, could see into the human psyche. And, also like Joe, she was no slouch at motivating others.

With that advice, Clara's insight, and our desperate need, I rethought my approach. Instead of offering Romana a job—run the new gym, an obvious comedown for an artist—I needed to convince her we would create a state-of-the art studio that would be hers. The new Pilates would be her stage, and she would have an important role in the world of dance. She would be the woman who saved Joe's work, preserved his memory, and most importantly, revitalized the essence of Joe's Contrology. I recast Romana as hero, as savior: the new Queen of Pilates. I even visualized her in the costume of royalty, wearing a diamond-and-platinum crown.

After rehearsing my new approach until it sounded spontaneous, I called Romana and said I had a new idea that I thought might interest her. "Could we meet one more time?" She agreed to another coffee—a very good sign. At our second meeting, I suggested that I had misread what I thought she wanted. I told her we didn't want an employee any more than she wanted to be one. We wanted a dynamic, commanding figure to carry on with Joe's work, bring it up to date, and move it into the future. I presented a word picture to her, painting her role in the new venture as the Queen of Pilates, Joe's protégée, successor, and savior.

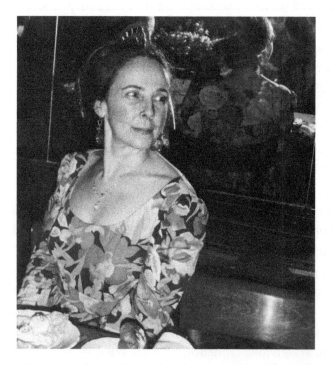

Romana Kryzanowska at Clara Pilates's ninetieth birthday party, 1971.

Romana stepped into the story I created for her and brought it to life, like a great actress stepping into a Dior gown for her walk on the red carpet. I put into her head her uniqueness, her exceptionalism, her vital role in the unfolding story of Pilates. It fell on fertile soil. She began to ask questions: "Would I be the boss?"

"Yes."

"Would anyone tell me what to teach or how to teach?"

"There is no one that could, except Clara, and I know she won't."

"Do I alone decide on hours, helpers, and things like that?"

"Of course."

"What about you? Are you my boss?"

"No, but I want to work with you on the financial management to see that we have enough money and stuff like that."

"Okay, I will need help with that."

It was such a wonderful story I created with the passion only desperation can produce that Romana wrapped it around herself as if I had discovered her true purpose, her destiny.

If anything saved Joe's work and legacy, Romana's willingness to take over was it. And we, the members of 939 Studio Corp., were so happy to have her, and to get back to just going to the studio (it was no longer a gym), we gave her free rein and half of the ownership. With one exception insisted upon by Romana and the investors: I had to supervise the business side, set up accounts and procedures, and at least once a week meet with Romana and review operations and accounts. I was delighted to do it. I thought I might come to like Romana. She was a bundle of energy and enthusiasm and had a feisty quality that appealed to me.

With Romana on board, and a spanking new studio, Contrology started a whole new life. That life tested whether it had the inherent ability to survive, or whether Contrology required Joe. Joe had thought the magic was the system. We worried that it was the man, not the system. Romana was the key: everything fell on her shoulders because there was no one else.

The studio was now just off Fifth Avenue on West 56th Street. It occupied the top floor of a converted brownstone. Designed by our committee to meet our needs, the space became the prototype for modern Pilates studios. Not that we had much choice, squeezing it into a narrow but deep space in an old brownstone. With its clean white décor, mirrored walls, rubber-tiled floors, a reception desk, and a prominent bronze bust of Joe watching over all of us, it was sharp, contemporary, and very attractive. The old-world look favored by Joe was left behind on Eighth Avenue.

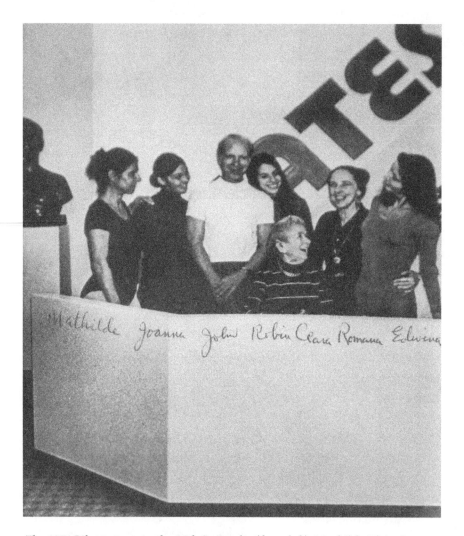

The 1974 Pilates team in the 56th St. Studio (from left): Mathilde Klein, Joanna, John Winters, Robin, Clara Pilates, Romana Kryzanowska, Edwina Fontaine.

Gone, too, was the European influence. No Oriental carpets, no photos on the wall, just pure working the body: community sweating. Even the apparatus was all new. The Reformers, the dominant piece of equipment, were all made of brushed aluminum with black upholstery, chromed springs, and belting-leather straps. The foot bars were no longer bent plumbing pipes but beautifully welded aluminum tubing. No mahogany or claw feet allowed in this spanking new environment. Even the apparatus Joe made, like the Ladder Barrel, the Cadillac, the Chair, and the Guillotine, were all spiffed up, and the wood polished to look good in the new contemporary world of Pilates. Pilates had morphed from a gym to a studio. This, all by itself, was a game changer.

It was both an abrupt change and a continuation. The basics continued with only slight detours here and there. Clara was still occasionally looking over the operation, but from a farther distance and from a position of powerlessness. She might discreetly offer a suggestion to Romana, and Romana might relay Clara's correction to a customer while Clara was still there, but Romana was now chief choreographer and orchestra conductor all in one. Pilates was in her hands. Romana could make of it what she wanted. She was free of Joe; all that was left was in the muscle memory of less than fifty students and a few instructors, all of whom were now under her care and her control. The freedom that Romana was accorded resulted in a vital change: the ability of an instructor to alter or amend or supplement or ignore sacred choreography. Fortunately, we had found the one person who could fill the job requirement, and she was brilliant.

We were in swanky town, just off Fifth Avenue, a block from Tiffany's, Bergdorf Goodman, Bonwit Teller, and back-to-back with Bendel. If location was important to our clientele, we were where they were. Contrary to the pejorative "designed by committee," our committee had done a superb job with the new studio. It had a reception desk and real locker rooms. Romana even had a small, private office opening into the main room, which, because it was long and narrow, allowed the equipment to be grouped by routine. Reformers were still front and center as Joe had them. We had location, environment, a good product, and management. All we needed were our old clients to continue and a regular supply of new clients. With just a little more business we would cover the salaries, the rent, and the other maintenance expenses.

We and Romana had high hopes. In the almost twenty-five years since the end of World War II, and the intervention of two smaller wars, Korea and Vietnam, people had let themselves go to pot. Diabetes, obesity, cardiac problems, bad backs, and cancer were on the rise. Regular, vigorous exercise had become accepted as a necessary health benefit. Svelte, nimble bodies were the rage, not only for appearance, not only to flatter women in bikinis and miniskirts, not only to be able to dance all night at clubs, but because it was an indispensable element of style. Running became popular. The New York City Marathon was first run in 1970, with fifty-five finishers and probably one hundred spectators. (Now it has over fifty thousand finishers and millions of spectators.)

Studio 54 opened in New York in 1977. Aerobics became a craze in the early 1980s. Pilates, little changed since Joe started teaching it in the late 1920s, was not the exercise program society was seeking. It remained tightly tied to routines very different from the fat burning, calorie gulping, drug and alcohol purging that the Studio 54 adherents and all their wannabes were looking for. Nothing in Pilates resembled what dancers were doing in rock videos or at the clubs. Pilates was closer to the *Nutcracker* than to disco. The new world of exercise was focused on plenty of sweat; rapid, repetitive movement; deafening music; and an instructor auditioning for a part in *Chorus Line*. "No pain, no gain" was the mantra.

Aerobics was the primary popular activity marked by rapid continuous movement in classes ranging from a few to sometimes one hundred people. Aerobics demanded exertion to the max, inspired or propelled by very loud and ear-damaging music and super-energetic instructors wearing a headset and shrieking over the music. The activity required moving everything on your body that could be moved. You were a slacker if at the end of your session you weren't sweaty and breathless, carrying a soaked towel, gulping water. A whole industry came into being just to supply the wet wipes to disinfect the floor, or the mats, or the boards everyone stood on. The rooms themselves were hot and stinky, and that was considered to be a good thing. We were all atoning for the abuses in our diet and drinking habits and perhaps rather sketchy lifestyles. Our confessional was this brightly lit, smelly room filled with all sorts of bodies jumping, leaping, bending, stepping, and breathing hard to rock-and-roll rhythms and screaming instructions. Stretching was done for a few moments at the beginning and a few moments at the end but not to stretch or tone, only to warm up for and cool down from the rigors of the class.

Pounds were shed, buttocks firmed up, legs became defined, and the bodies, pumped as they were with endorphins and adrenaline, exhibited marked changes. People learned the moves, learned how to step up and stay balanced on little platforms. It was competitive. At first you watched and worked to keep up. Trying to hear the instructor over the pounding music was a challenge. Eventually when you learned the steps and could visually interpret the instructions, you mindlessly followed along. The hotshots needed to be in the front row. There were those who did it twice a day. It was Bollywood on steroids and addictive as hell. For a while you felt better and looked better. You had a sense of accomplishment. You came clean. You purged. You made room for more abuse. It was fun, it was social, and it was sexy. Entire lines of clothing were designed for aerobics: body wicking, stink preventing, loose fitting but flattering. Sweatbands were essential, aerobic shoes helpful, and high-impact absorbing socks de rigueur.

All through the 1980s, aerobics was not only attracting all kinds of people who had never participated in organized physical activity unrelated to playing a sport, but it was cutting into the barely surviving customer base of the Pilates studio. Aerobics was not competing with Pilates—the aerobics world didn't even know about Pilates. Simply put, Pilates was not on the radar of those looking for a quick exercise fix during the course of the day. Our exercise-addicted potential customer base was headed to gyms, athletic clubs, Ys where classes, some of them quite large, assembled frequently. And some of those participants were formerly Pilates clients who now abandoned it for the endorphin high of aerobics, not to mention the mindlessness of simply imitating rapid dance moves.

Aerobics did provide one leg of what Joe had referred to as the three-legged stool of healthy living: regular exercise. And it attracted the trendsetters and the celebrities, media stars, and the society-column inhabitants. And where the socially anointed beautiful people go, so, too, go the press, the publicity folks, the imitators and emulators, the hip, and then the rest of society. A mass movement toward group exercise was underway, but it headed toward high-exertion, vigorous activity, quick fixes, and little regard for the workings of the body: the opposite direction from Pilates. The "new exercise" mocked the lengthy learning curve of Pilates and the slow development of the mind-body connection. With the shift to speed, sweat, and the endorphin rush, the little life left in Pilates was close to extinction. Its practitioners diminished through attrition, but at least those who remained were unshakable.

Some of us, and I was one, tried aerobics. It was fun, a great sweat, an opportunity if one stood in the back as I did, to help time pass and mask the discomfort by focusing on a lady in front shaking her tightly clad booty. But it was not Pilates. It had nothing to do with gaining control over your body and its movements. It had nothing to do with concentrating on your muscles. It was not about stretching and flexibility and range of motion and enhancing your everyday movement. And while I felt good after aerobics—sometimes because it was over, and I hadn't stumbled or fallen laughably behind—I never felt reinvigorated and relaxed as I did after doing Pilates. Certainly, everyone left aerobics with pink cheeks and some energy in the tank, but no one left standing taller and straighter with an easy, relaxed gait. Mostly after aerobics I wanted a nap. Not so after Pilates. I was energized.

It turned out that aerobics was also dangerous in a very sneaky and subtle way. The collateral damage was significant. It, like tooth decay, just took a long time to show up. While your muscles were firming, your skin was aging. While your body fat was disappearing, so, too, was the fat under the skin on your face, leaving your face looking older, wrinkled, and a bit worn out. While your cardio capacity and your oxygen efficiency were certainly improving, your tendons and ligaments were stiffening, and you were losing flexibility. True, you might leave a really good aerobics session with a postcoital glow, having stared for nearly an hour at the leader, a really cute person of—back then—one or the other genders, with great buns and super moves, but you also left with sore knees and sometimes a creaky lower back. Not unexpected results from pounding on a hard floor for forty-five minutes. But these were subtle impairments that you certainly could work through, so you thought, and well worth the benefits and pleasures of aerobics classes. That is, until your joints hurt so bad you couldn't keep up in class.

Because aerobics was a time bomb for your joints, and because repeating the same steps over and over without any real sense of challenge or mastery was boring, it had a limited life span. When it got boring, or when joints began to hurt, or when you couldn't take the noise anymore, Pilates moved into position as the antidote. Pilates put people back together. It didn't stress your joints, and it significantly improved your body, providing many of the same benefits of aerobics without the damage. Once the attraction to aerobics wore off, during the late 1980s, and society was programmed to exercise, Pilates came into focus. So aerobics was ironically one of several forces that saved Pilates from its second near-death experience by creating the need for exercise.

Even though Romana's Pilates routine closely followed Joe's prescription, other important changes crept in with Romana's management. Right from the beginning, she took over as the master teacher. Romana kept John Winters and Hannah Sakamirda—she had to; they were the only ones who knew all the customers and the routine for each apparatus. Romana instituted an intern program and attracted young ballet students, hers mostly, to assist and to learn the routines. No one had a private session with Romana, although she did have her favorites (and her unfavorites). In addition, Romana's daughter Sari Mejia Santos helped. And with several ballet students there as interns "on scholarship," as Romana would say, no one suffered from a lack of attention.

There were many times when I came to the studio, either to work out or review our finances, when there were more scholarship students than customers. The interns were of two basic types: 1) those who were genuinely interested in Pilates and put the customer first and 2) those who were genuinely interested in themselves and their dancing career and put themselves first. The latter caused huge resentment from the clients, particularly when they occupied equipment that the client was waiting to use. Many of us wondered whether these ballet dancers were actually helping in the studio or just continuing their dance education with Romana. When I tried to talk to her about our concerns, I was met with "That is for me, and only me, to decide." Romana was formidable, born to be a diva. She was intransigent—even threatened to quit—when we had a conflict. The test came over her dogs.

Romana had two large, white Afghan hounds. They were beautiful, regal animals and drew considerable attention as she walked them the mile between her apartment and the studio. I thought they made Romana look short and a bit dumpy, as they were tall and frighteningly thin with ribs showing prominently. They were also indifferent to people, although well-behaved and docile. They looked like ornamental dogs and in Romana's case were leash candy. She brought the dogs into the studio, and they would spend the day in her little back office. They took up almost all the floor space there. Now and then one of them would wander into the exercise area and poke around the clients. The dog was not looking for affection or attention. He/she (I never knew) needed to get up and roam about to break the monotony of his or her confinement. Romana would order the beast back to jail.

From time to time I got complaints. They came from several sources: people who didn't like dogs in the studio for whatever reason, people who loved dogs and didn't like the idea that these specimens were confined to close quarters for such long periods, and people who saw the dog as a dangerous, movable obstacle. I would ask the complainers if they had spoken to Romana. Several had and she had listened, nodded, and ignored them. Even our investors had complained, to no effect. I was told she was abrupt and rude. Several clients had not complained out of fear of angering the goddess. No question; I had to talk to Romana.

When I brought the issue up to her, Romana dismissed me with "This is my studio and the customers will just have to get used to it." I contacted a few investors, and we decided to ban the animals. We were now facing a constitutional crisis. What would we do if Romana dug in her heels—which I knew she would? I looked forward to this confrontation like I would a root canal.

The meeting went far worse than I'd expected. I tried to be diplomatic, suggesting that I was not the only one who objected to the dogs. The investors were concerned. One of them suggested that if their presence cost us one customer, that was enough to ban them. Romana never said a word. She put the leashes on the dogs, put on her coat, and with chin held high and fire in her eyes, rang for the elevator and walked out.

Fortunately, we had several assistants in the studio at the time. And, equally fortunately, they didn't believe the dogs should be there. Even the ballet dancers, who all treated Romana like a minor deity, agreed to help cover for her, and we got through the day without a hitch. The next morning, I arranged to open the studio, fully expecting another confrontation with the Queen of the Animals and her two royal canine appendages, but she didn't come in. Hasty arrangements were made to staff the studio, and I departed for my law office, which was just a few blocks away. I left word to call me when Romana arrived. That call did not come. We were able to stumble along during an indeterminate cold war. We needed the boss; she needed to be there. After all, she was a 50 percent partner, and this was her pedestal.

After about a week, Romana returned without the dogs. She never said a word about them and never brought them to the studio, at least when I was there.

When it came to the exercises, Romana was detail oriented, extremely helpful to everyone, and perceptive. She, like Joe, could fix people and give them specific exercises to remedy physical problems. She even diagnosed me as having shingles. The ballet dancers and the Afghan hounds were small blips on the big picture, so it was easy to ignore stuff like that and remain grateful for her presence.

With our spiffy new gym, spiffy fashion soon followed. Gone was the old-world look. Clara's sanitarium nurse look no longer worked. Our ballet-dancer interns were very body conscious, and their outfits reflected their profession: tending toward tights, leg warmers, and leotards. The paying customers were not to be outshone by the young dancers/interns, so the women adopted dancer outfits, adding here and there bright colors and attempts at originality.

Looking well-dressed while exercising was not of any concern in Joe's time. Quite to the contrary: Joe wanted everyone in a mock uniform to avoid distraction and "clothes envy." Perhaps, with Joe not there to impose his notions of propriety in the gym, and his disdain of exercise as an act of vanity, clients finally could acknowledge they exercised to look good, and they wanted to look good when they exercised. Joe certainly cared about his appearance, wearing as little as possible to exhibit his remarkable physique and vitality.

New people did trickle in, mostly through word of mouth from existing customers. When a new prospect arrived, Romana was far better at keeping them than Joe, which is saying very little, because he was so bad at it. Nevertheless, the retention rate was low. One look when the studio was busy said it all: This was work. Pilates was at that time not for everyone.

With the spiffy gym, the omnipresent ballet dancers, and the introduction of fashion into workout clothes, the gym of Joe's day transitioned from masculine to feminine. And the exercises acquired more than a trace of ballet. Romana began to change Joe's natural positions to what she considered more "beautiful" positions. When Romana demonstrated an exercise, her posture and movement reflected her long years of ballet. Most of our gang of old-timers ignored these changes, but the ballet-dancer interns and the new customers were learning a revised, and less natural, choreography.

From the day the studio opened, we raised the price for a session from Joe's "give me five dollars" to seven dollars, and we kept track of payments. Not yet had the idea struck of significantly increasing the price per session and then selling multiple sessions at a discount. It could be the investor group didn't want to pay more for their sessions. Or we were not sufficiently businesslike.

Romana slowly and subtly changed the "come at your convenience" feature that had caused attendance bubbles on Eighth Avenue. Everyone who wanted or needed Romana's attention made an appointment to arrive at a specified time. It did get crowded at the usual hours, although with the location in the heart of New York's prime shopping area, many customers came during slow periods. During the busy times, Romana was everywhere and flitted around the studio more like a dog trainer with a large unruly class than a ballet teacher. She paid some attention to everyone, much more to those who made appointments.

Romana assigned her young ballet interns to assist specific customers. That relieved her of having to be everywhere at once and gave the customer a personal touch. The assignment was informal, and the customer received a good deal of help adjusting springs, putting feet into the straps, and so forth, but very little instruction or correction. This was the start of private sessions for certain customers. Not everyone had their own minder. The ugly face of "teacher's pets" entered the picture. The notion of a hierarchy of favorites was new, not at all something Joe would do or abide, and, if you were not in the chosen category, disturbing. With hierarchy comes competition, in the form of kissing up, but Romana seemed oblivious. She, I suspect, was accustomed to dancers seeking favorable treatment: another carryover from ballet, which is highly competitive.

Pilates, when I learned it, wasn't competitive. Sure, everyone wanted to be on Joe's good side, if there was such a thing. But it didn't matter. There were no benefits. He treated everyone the same. Joe Pilates did not have a kiss-up bone in his body. I am sure he had favorites deep down. If he did, he hid it. Nor was he starstruck by celebrity or status. Everyone was corrected, pushed, and reprimanded equally. Joe's indifference to status or celebrity was refreshing and set the tone throughout his gym. No one made a fuss about a celebrity.

Such was not the case with Romana. While it was great to be one of her obvious favorites, and there were many, it was not so good to be out of favor. If you were in favor, you got her attention. She worked with you, corrected you, and assigned one of her better interns to you. There was still no chitchat, no personal stuff, although Romana, unlike Joe, could turn on the charm and make someone feel special.

Romana's obvious preference for certain clients was picked up by her protégées, and they, too, paid more attention to the favorites. Tension developed. I got complaints. New clients felt like outsiders. Old customers felt neglected: some dropped out. Romana, in choosing favorites, placed much more emphasis on the connection to the dance world or even status as some sort of celebrity. Sam Waterston, a prominent actor, was treated extremely well, while right next to him a very successful manufacturer, or someone connected to the fashion world, or a college professor, or just an ordinary client was ignored. This was bad for business.

We coasted along no more stable than we had been during the years after Joe's death. Yet, when you were in the studio, and it was bustling, and you could hear Romana's enthusiasm, it was hard to believe we were barely self-sustaining. I had the sense that the business was on a mild downhill slope. There were long quiet stretches between the morning crowd and the folks who came at lunch hour, and another quiet stretch between lunch hour and the after-work crowd. This was tough on Romana. We were not attracting new business, and as I went over the books weekly, that was ominous.

While the exercise world outside our doors was blossoming over the ten-year period since we'd moved, Pilates was languishing. And for much the same reasons as it had under Joe. It was locked into a rigid method, taught and controlled by a rigid individual. It was just a different rigidity. To maintain control, Romana avoided allowing others in. Just like with Joe, no successors were being trained. There was no impetus to establish branch studios or to market the 56th Street operation.

The working group and the executive committee of Julie, my dad, and me had pretty much stepped away and lost interest in anything to do with managing the studio. We had achieved our objective: We had a studio for ourselves that seemed to be self-sustaining, Clara was taken care of, and Romana really didn't need or even want us anymore. No one expected a return on their investment. It was enough they had a place to exercise and they were not asked to invest additional money. Or worry about sustainability.

The working group, the executive committee, even the investors reverted to being clients, now with the limited benefits of being favorites. It was easy to overlook the slow drumbeat warning us that history was about to repeat itself. After all, the fewer the customers, the better it was for us—less competition for the equipment and more attention from Romana and the assistants. Pilates, while still alive, remained in the Dark Ages but now in modern dress. It was not a new Pilates, just a different Pilates.

After ten years of lurching along in the 56th Street studio, neither advancing nor crumbling, Romana appeared tired and ready to throw in the towel. She was taking more and more time off; her usual enthusiastic voice and personal energy were down. The change in Romana brought several of us out of hibernation. I was contacted by some of the old-timers with complaints and concerns. I set up another meeting and once again invited our regular customers and Romana. Romana told us that the operation had deteriorated from slightly above the cusp of failure to frequently sinking below it. She said she had done her best to enlist new clients, but the interest wasn't there. She admitted she was tired of running the studio, but that she still loved the work. Everyone at the meeting agreed with Romana; it was time to let it go. We had done our best, but we were not covering costs.

In June 1984, we planned to close the doors and walk away. We didn't have anything to sell. Then, just as the ax was about to fall, a savior appeared: a very dedicated client named Lari Stanton. Stanton was the president of his family's business, founded in 1906, a well-known glove manufacturer, Aris Isotoner. When Romana told Stanton that we were preparing to close shop, Lari was terribly upset. Working out at the studio had been his early morning routine for many years, and he felt he couldn't live without it. Without blinking an eye, he said his company would buy it, proving it's good to be president. Lari, who many a morning was next to me on a Reformer, met with me and we negotiated a price of $100,000, which would give Romana for her 50 percent about $50,000 (a substantial amount of money back then) and the investors a 30 percent return on their capital contributions. This was pure charity on Stanton's part, mostly out of his affection for Romana. On paper we had negligible value. The equipment, the lease, the fixtures had value only for a going business. We were a going-out-of-business business. The Aris corporate staff would take over my job and some of Romana's; she would be an employee of the new owner, with reduced hours and no business or administrative duties. That Pilates would continue to have a home greatly softened the blow to me and the few investors still dedicated to the program. Some of us thought this was a positive move. Good thought, but it would turn out to be wrong.

When we had moved to 56th Street in 1972, our investor group and Romana had the chutzpah to believe we could turn a failing mom-and-pop business into a healthy, self-sustaining enterprise. Either Lari Stanton had to know this was not a business, or he was smitten with magic dust. His staid, old family company, manufacturing one quality product, wasn't equipped to reverse our fifteen-year tradition of hanging on by the fingernails. I knew that Stanton was doing this act of charity for personal reasons, but I negotiated as if it were smart business. I had an obligation to Romana and the investors.

After ownership changed, my relationship with the Pilates studio and Romana faded to zero. There was nothing that kept us together any longer. I was busy with my own life and not at all sad about leaving behind this strange, vague avocation.

Romana continued to live as the Queen of Pilates claiming, falsely, that the crown was placed on her head by Joe himself. Instead, it came from a desperate lawyer seducing her to take a job that no one else wanted. She bought the fantastical sales pitch that I invented purely out of necessity to obtain her services as the last possibility for keeping Joe's work alive. She altered her history with Joe from mere young student to intimate family friend; she asserted that her version of Contrology was Joe's version, which she claimed was bequeathed to her. She installed herself as the heiress; the one true voice, the anointed disciple.

And it was good she filled that role and grew into it. Never mind that her history with Joe was as a very young dancer with a physical problem, and the exercises that she learned differed greatly from the basic Contrology that everyone did in the gym. She quickly learned and then mastered the routines through the patience and goodwill of Joe's former assistants, John Winters and Mathilde Klein, a former student of Joe's who returned to the new studio as a teacher.

As a dancer, the choreography was easy for Romana. As a former ballet teacher, she knew how to motivate and inspire. Romana was a gifted and inspiring teacher. And like the true artist she was, she added her interpretations. I, and our whole group, supported her to the hilt because Pilates needed a take-charge, dominating person. And that was Romana. Convincing Romana to step into Joe's shoes was among the most important steps in perpetuating Pilates.

We, the new company, had accomplished our goal and created a new Pilates. We thought we had continued Joe's work and had been fully faithful to it. We were correct about the "continued" part but not the "faithful" part. Romana proved Pilates could exist without Joe. Modifications could occur. She proved someone other than Joe could teach and manage and satisfy Joe's long-term clients. Romana, by establishing herself as the leader of Pilates, by proving that Pilates could continue without Joe, was crucial to its growth and expansion. It was a first, a true breakthrough. We had handed it over to someone who saw the essence of Pilates and had the talent, and the courage, to introduce her interpretations into the strict choreography insisted upon by Joe. Romana broke the chain of rigidity he had imposed on Contrology. She had a different version of the one true way. After all, she believed that Joe ordained her to do exactly that.

Throughout the rest of her life, Romana insisted that her version of Pilates was the one and true way, and those who taught what they claimed to be Pilates were imposters, revisionists, plagiarists, phonies, and misguided souls. Unless, and this is a big unless, they had graduated from Romana's intensive training program and she had certified them as teachers.

If a New Yorker wanted to do Pilates, Romana was almost your only choice. Her monopoly on the proper practice of Pilates was easy to enforce when she took over in 1972, because except for a few other small very private studios, no one was there to challenge her. Starting in the early 1990s, or maybe before, when others with her talent and drive wanted to make a career of teaching or having a studio, Romana's monopoly crumbled. Many of those new entries into studio ownership or teaching were trained by Romana. Once they thoroughly absorbed the essentials of Pilates, as Romana required, they applied their own ideas and approaches to teaching it and dealing with clients. That, to claimed purists like Romana, was heresy; to others it was revolutionary and exciting.

Joe had to reinvent himself to survive in New York. He had to shed his own history and replace it with one palatable to Americans. He not only had to leave home and change countries, language, and cultures, he had to abandon his history—the unchangeable facts of his prior existence. Throughout his lifetime, he hid his past and inhabited the story of himself that he developed. He was like a stage actor, playing a very intense character, who can never, even for a moment, whether onstage or off, step out of character and be himself. From my time with him, I believe he was successful in becoming his adopted identity.

The odd thing is that Joe lived the last half of his life playing an invented part, Romana did the very same thing. Maybe she didn't have to do it as a matter of survival as Joe was compelled to do, but once she adopted her new self, she stayed with it. And it worked for the business. Role-playing served both Joe and Romana professionally, but what did it do to the rest of their lives?

On August 14, 1984, the assets of 939 Studio Corp. were sold to Aris Isotoner. My involvement ended. Aris Isotoner kept the flame burning for a little over two years, and on December 10, 1986, it sold the assets to an instructor named Wei-Tai Hom. He kept the doors open for a little longer than two more years. On April 1, 1989, Pilates ended its sixty-three-year New York residence, although Romana continued to teach it privately elsewhere.

But the seeds of a new Pilates were germinating far away.

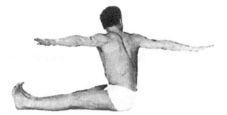

CHAPTER 7

Starting Anew: The Western Renaissance of Pilates

In the years while the New York studio and Romana were striving to gain a toehold in the exercise industry, Pilates was taking root in the western United States. As is typical of New Yorkers, none of us in New York City paid attention to the goings-on west of the Hudson River. Out west, well below Manhattan's radar, former New Yorkers were successfully pursuing careers as Pilates teachers. Active studios were popping up in Santa Fe; Seattle; and Boulder and Denver, Colorado, in addition to the Ron Fletcher Studio on Wilshire Boulevard in the heart of Beverly Hills. Ron Fletcher, in particular, was to have a profound effect on the survival and future of Pilates.

I knew about Ron Fletcher because I worked with Clara to set him up in business. That happened right after we opened our new studio on 56th Street, in 1972. I was having my regular dinner with Clara, sitting on one of the Wunda Chairs in her apartment, when she told me about a man, an excellent dancer, who had been a student of Joe's. Ron Fletcher had visited her a few days earlier. She said she hadn't seen him in many years, and he looked terrible. I was happy to have a story, and I particularly liked these little trips back in time. Clara told me about his dancing career, which ended in the 1950s. According to Clara, after he couldn't dance, he worked as a freelance choreographer until he was hired to choreograph and direct a dance for a famous ice-skating company. He found that strange because he had never ice-skated, but they liked what he had done for a Broadway show and thought he could do something fresh for ice-skaters. He took the commission, and everyone loved the ice dancing, so she said. Then they asked him if he would work full-time for them choreographing and directing all their shows and traveling around the world with them. Clara said Ron was very proud of his part in the success of the Ice Capades: they paid him a lot of money and treated him like a star. The skaters loved his work, the audience loved the performances, and he became famous.

Clara said, "He was too famous because it went to his head. He spent lots of money, began to drink too much, eat too much, and use drugs." Clara's voice carried both her disapproval and her empathy. She stated, in a troubled voice, that alcohol took over his life, and eventually he was fired after he was too drunk to choreograph and too drunk to direct. "Ron told me he was in AA, and after being sober for a few years, he wanted to come back to the gym and get in shape and figure out what to do with his life. He said he was thinking about moving to Los Angeles. He said he still had a little money."

Clara turned the conversation from Fletcher's story to hers. "I remember when he came to Joe a few years after the war. Martha Graham sent him, I believe. He had something the matter with his ankle or his leg, and Joe fixed him up. He loved the work and came almost every day for several years. I worked with him mostly because Joe was very impatient with homosexual men who were show-offs and very feminine like Ron. And Ron wanted special—actually undivided—attention, and Joe didn't do that. Ron liked me, and back then, before he became an alcoholic,

he would come occasionally to have a beer or bring wine. He was an excellent student and learned the routine quickly. Like all dancers he did the exercises perfectly, and Joe even told me that Ron had a very good understanding of his body, and great control and coordination." So I suggested to Ron that he should open a Pilates studio.

Clara said he mentioned he was moving to California. She thought that was a great idea, a great place for Pilates, and told him so. Fletcher said he knew lots of people in the dance world there, and a few celebrities, and he would think about opening a Pilates studio there. He agreed a California studio was a good idea; something he could do and might even enjoy. Then, Clara told me that he called and said he liked my idea and wanted to work something out with the New York studio, and he would pay us if we could help get the equipment.

Clara continued: "I wanted to help but I thought I had better get Romana's and your permission because you and your people were in charge. So yesterday when I was over at the new place, I asked Romana. She said no. She wanted no one teaching a different version of Pilates, it was hard enough keeping everything pure, and she had no idea who he was or if he could be trusted or what he might do in Los Angeles."

Then, Clara got to the point: "I want you to help him if you can and your people agree. You are good at getting Romana to go along."

I told Clara a West Coast Pilates studio might work. It was partly selfish, as I, too, wanted to branch out. I thought it might be good for our clients (like me) who went to Los Angeles and vice versa. And if a movie star came to visit us in New York, that would attract publicity.

I talked to several of our investor group members. Everyone in the group had a soft heart for Clara, and if she liked this fellow, Ron Fletcher, we had to honor her. The most important thing to three members of the group was giving Clara a paying job. These three members had been supporting Clara since Joe's death, to the tune of about $5,000 a month. While for the three that sum was not significant, Clara felt bad about having to take it as charity. The investors wanted me to convince Romana to go along with the Ron Fletcher studio idea and negotiate a deal with him to "employ" Clara as a consultant to help him teach the way Joe did. The fee to Clara was set at $5,000 a month. So once again

I had the troublesome mission of convincing an equal but intransigent partner to do something she had already rejected.

For this task I took my time developing a negotiating strategy. I thought of three arguments that might work: 1) Romana had affection and respect for Clara, 2) an LA branch might help our business in New York, and 3) Romana, not the studio, could be the supplier of the Pilates equipment to Fletcher and thereby receive a commission.

I met Romana for dinner after the studio closed for the evening, in a trendy Italian restaurant in the same building the studio occupied. After we sat down, ordered our food, and were sipping a split of fine champagne, I said: "Romana, I want to talk to you about Ron Fletcher. I am speaking on behalf of Clara and our investors. I know you told Clara no, but I don't think Clara gave you the full story. There are several reasons why I think this is a good deal for us, for you, and for Clara."

I had her attention but noticed that ever so slight stiffening of her back. Romana, like all good dancers, communicated with her body. Fortunately, she stayed in listening mode—she didn't look away, bored—as I went through my arguments for working with Fletcher. Kaboom! She liked the idea. We finished our pasta, dessert, coffee, and wine talking about other things, even gossiping about our clients, always a favorite topic of ours.

Once again, I moved Romana from no to yes. I called Fletcher and told him: "You have been approved by Clara and Romana to open a studio in California. Romana will help. Let's get it on paper." He said fine. I drew up a simple agreement giving him a license to identify his work as Joseph Pilates's Contrology, obligating him to stick to Joe's routine, engaging Clara as a consultant required to visit monthly for quality control, and paying her $5,000 per month. Fletcher honored that commitment until her death in 1976 at ninety-three. And Romana started a substantial side business supplying Pilates equipment not only to Fletcher but to many others.

Clara conveniently forgot about her obligation to visit the Beverly Hills Fletcher Studio for quality control. After Fletcher was up and running for several months, I reminded Clara of this commitment and arranged to take her to see Fletcher's operation. I bought airplane tickets and reserved two rooms in the Beverly Wilshire Hotel, catty-corner from Fletcher's studio. As our departure time approached, Romana told me Clara was very nervous about the trip. Clara didn't think she was up to it because of her age and very poor eyesight. But she didn't want to upset me. When I asked Clara directly, she told me she didn't think she was strong enough, and she didn't want to inter-fere in Fletcher's business. She trusted him.

I thought it would be good for her to go and get out of her apart-ment, and I knew she was strong enough. She had no trouble walking the three long blocks to the studio. I tried again: "Maybe Ron wants you to make sure he is teaching the way Joe would have wanted. And you have an obligation from the agreement."

That didn't work. She said she was confident Ron would excuse her from coming all that way. She then allowed, "I don't want to inconve-nience you, but I think you should check on him just so he knows we care."

"If it is okay with Ron that I go alone, I will make the trip. But you have to call and find out if it is okay just to send me."

A few days later she told me she had called him. He was disap-pointed she couldn't come because she would like the studio, but it was okay to send me.

I had not met Fletcher face-to-face. When I called to make a date to visit his studio, he was standoffish. I couldn't pin him down for a time and didn't want to make that expensive trip to be jerked around. So, I asked him if I could sign up for a session. He agreed.

He was to be the instructor. When I arrived, right on time, he took one look at me, asked if I was okay on my own, said he wouldn't charge me, and showed me to a Reformer. Then he left me alone to do my thing while he buzzed about teaching the few others in the studio, checking on me occasionally. The studio was in a superb location on the second floor of a typical Beverly Hills low-profile office building. Back in the early days of Fletcher's studio, he taught the routine just as Joe had taught it to all of us. From what I saw and heard as I was doing the routine, Fletcher taught enthusiastically. He was energetic and observant. And strict. People were moving at a good pace, but some of the movements were unusual although interesting. I was the only man there.

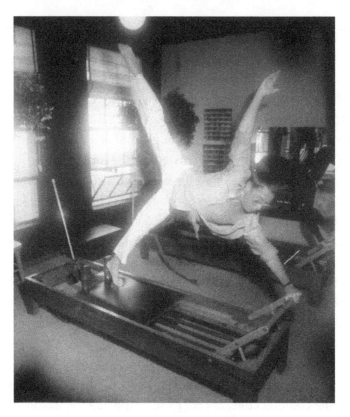

Ron Fletcher demonstrating "the Star," a very difficult and advanced position.

Joe and Fletcher both attracted celebrities. Fletcher turned it into publicity; Joe didn't. Fletcher wanted success and recognition. Joe hung on to one of his principles: Contrology would sell itself. Joe was not impressed by celebrities and probably didn't believe their endorsement could help him. Fletcher had the movie people: Raquel Welch, Candice Bergen, Cher, Barbra Streisand, Jane Fonda, and several other icons of the body beautiful. Fletcher knew their value to the business. Movie stars attracted much more attention and interest than the dance and opera people who went to Joe's. Times were different, as well. Once the gossip columnists, the celeb magazines, and the paparazzi got wind of stars exercising at Fletcher's, doing something called "Body Contrology," Fletcher was on the Hollywood map. He became a demi-celebrity. Even Nancy Reagan, who knew Fletcher from her acting days, dropped in for a Body Contrology exercise session. Fletcher, to protect his star clients from leering eyes as they exercised, installed around each Reformer those pull-around curtains you see in hospital rooms. Before the curtains, I can tell you from personal experience, it was extremely difficult to concentrate on my body when the body next to me belonged to Raquel Welch, which it did on my first visit.

Fletcher's use of the name "Body Contrology" was clever. The exercises had their roots in Joe's Contrology. Fletcher's movements varied somewhat, and he added additional routines of a basic nature. He was well-known for his "towel work." Fletcher's philosophy and basics were straight out of Pilates: symmetry, breath control, stretching, muscle awareness, and focus. The equipment was all of Joe's design, with the Reformer still center stage. Fletcher, nevertheless, sought to distance himself from Joe's Contrology. Body Contrology was different: a Fletcher invention. Fletcher, despite his flamboyance, was deadly serious as a teacher, and even though he was starstruck, he treated his celebrities sternly, insisting they do the hard work he demanded. They liked that. Not only had Fletcher moved to Los Angeles, so, too, had Pilates. The culture of Los Angeles informed, or as some might put it, infected, Pilates. Fletcher's was that typical seemingly oxymoronic combination of laid-back and serious. It was rigorous and fun. I, for one, thought it was great.

Back in New York, my verbal report to Clara and Romana was upbeat. I emphasized the energy, the enthusiasm, Fletcher's attention to detail. I skipped over the alterations in the routine and Fletcher's need for sole credit. I knew Clara and Romana would be disturbed to hear about variances from Joe's strict and pure Contrology. The LA influence was not something Clara and Romana needed to know about. I told them I enjoyed my session, that Fletcher was very busy teaching others as Joe had done, and that Joe's legacy (nonexistent at the time) was intact. From my vantage point I was happy to see Fletcher succeed so he could continue to pay Clara. I had no thoughts about whether he was good for Pilates.

In 1978, six years after he opened his Pilates space, Fletcher wrote a book, *Every Body Is Beautiful*, about his work, his studio, and mostly about his star clientele. The book mentions Joe and Clara once. There is no attribution of Fletcher's Body Contrology to the Contrology of Joe Pilates. There is no thank-you, no respect, nothing. The book is a mishmash of canned celebrity testimonials and photographs punctuated by Fletcher's sermonizing about breathing, learning your body, doing the movements (he deplores the word "exercise"). Joe and Clara would have been furious, and I can see Joe, had he been alive, grabbing his Walther PPK pistol and driving to LA and shooting Fletcher. I was revolted when I read the book. But not when I was in his studio. There was something okay about Fletcher putting his personal stamp on Pilates. But it was not okay to distance himself from Joe and Clara Pilates, the two people who made his success possible. Fletcher, as the fates would have it, would get an opportunity to redeem this lapse.

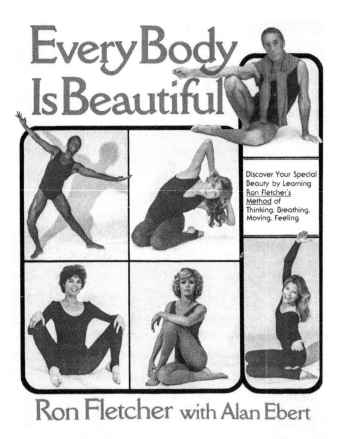

The cover of Ron's celebrity-studded book.

Fletcher firmly believed that the renaissance of Pilates, at least on the West Coast, was solely the product of his ability to attract and keep celebs. I never debated the point with him, but privately I disagreed. Fletcher underestimated his role by focusing on his celebrity appeal while ignoring the substance of what the celebs and everyone else came for: the Contrology of Joseph Pilates. The rebirth of Pilates took both Fletcher's ability to apply Joe's teaching and the celebrity of the people to whom it was applied. And none of this would have happened without these elements, as well as a substantial push from Clara. Fletcher lived to be ninety and was a beloved figure in the Pilates world when he died in 2011.

Fletcher did several other things that started Pilates on the road to rebirth. By establishing a studio in a place where no one ever heard of Contrology or Pilates, he showed others that to run a studio and teach Pilates, it wasn't necessary to be certified by Joe Pilates. Or to be in New York. Not everyone could open a studio and teach. It took study, aptitude, and practice, like so many other professions. But if you loved movement, loved helping others, and were attracted to Pilates, Fletcher demonstrated it was possible to make a living teaching it.

Fletcher broke through the rigidity of Joe's ironclad routine. He must have missed Joe's lecture on the unchangeability of the exercises or the routine, because he immediately began to improvise. Fletcher appreciated the basics of Contrology, but when he saw a better way to move the body, or an easier way, or a more enjoyable way, he felt free to change or augment the Pilates way. He respected and adopted the principles but not the choreography. That Fletcher wasn't bound by Joe's routine had to be expected: he was a very inventive choreographer and a dedicated student of movement.

Fletcher's freedom from slavish adherence to Joe's routines gave life to modern Pilates. It brought joy and creativity to the teaching. Who with any spirit or imagination would sign up to teach the exact same routine to everyone day after day?

Joe's routine needed an update; it needed to be brought into the current world of disco, modern dance, new music, and customers who wanted much more. Pilates, with its mystical power to survive, found just the person to jazz up Contrology, to add some variety and make it fun and hip. Pilates needed a showman, a choreographer, and a kinesiologist in one exuberant and energetic person and got it with Ron Fletcher.

The breakthrough into flexibility made Pilates attractive to teachers and students. Creative teachers could express themselves. Fletcher began a formal training program for prospective teachers early on, probably around 1975. Fletcher's students went out on their own, opening studios and centers in Boulder, Colorado; San Francisco; Santa Fe, New Mexico; and several other places. And as these studios opened, usually with one instructor, they were sought out due, in part, to the publicity attached to Pilates by the celebrities attending Fletcher's Beverly Hills studio. As they grew in popularity, the demand for teachers increased exponentially, and a burgeoning demand for equipment was created. The upward spiral had begun. The New Pilates of Fletcher's era, starting in right after he opened his studio in 1972, looked radically different from the one Joe left upon his death in 1967. It was young, vigorous, and pushed along by people inspired and taught by Ron Fletcher—two generations removed from Joseph Pilates.

In June 1983, Fletcher introduced Pilates to Dr. James Garrick, an orthopedic surgeon at St. Francis Hospital in San Francisco. Dr. Garrick was pioneering sports medicine as a specialty and saw the benefit of Pilates as an important tool for physical therapists. Right away Dr. Garrick, with Patricia Whiteside Norris, a former dancer, and Elizabeth Larkam, a master Pilates teacher, installed a Pilates program for rehabilitation therapy in the hospital, where it became a staple. And the hospital became a breeding ground to train other physical therapists as Pilates therapists. Finally Joe's mission of obtaining medical approval was accomplished.

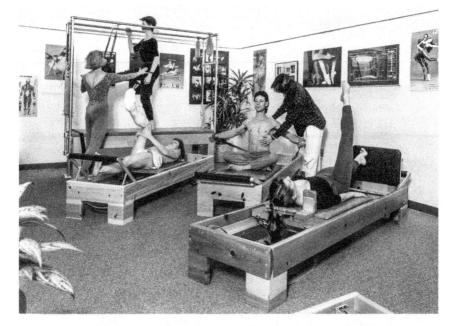

Physical therapy facility at St. Francis Hospital in San Francisco in 1984. Elizabeth Larkam, Balanced Body Master Trainer, is the therapist on the left, back to camera, assisting a patient on Joe's "Cadillac."

Barbara Huttner, a Fletcher Beverly Hills client and a wealthy lady who split her time between LA and Vail, Colorado, wanted Fletcher to come to Vail for a week, teach clients just as he did in Beverly Hills, and also "train" a few "personal trainers" to teach in Vail after he went home. Ms. Huttner needed her Pilates. Fletcher was reluctant; he didn't believe in training. He said: "One trains animals but teaches humans." Fletcher's hesitancy was overmatched by her persuasive powers, reputed to be near irresistible. Ms. Huttner prevailed and lured Fletcher to Vail for a week of very intensive work. Thanks to her, Fletcher as the teacher of teachers gave birth to the Pilates "workshop," which is the mainstay of Pilates continuing education to this day.

By expanding Pilates in these ways, Fletcher created a demand for equipment. He started with equipment that Clara or Romana sold to him. He then began sourcing the equipment locally and commissioned a Hollywood set designer to make a Reformer. The Reformer was based on plans probably taken from the Reformers made for the new studio back in 1972. They were fabricated by Donald Gratz with aluminum bases. Clara had the plans and gave them to Fletcher. The set designer charged Fletcher $3,000—cheap by today's standards but expensive then, the same price as a new VW Beetle.

In the late 1970s, as Fletcher expanded and needed more equipment, two of his movie star clients, Natalie Wood and Robert Wagner, introduced him to a waterbed maker to the stars in Los Angeles named Ken Endelman. Fletcher had lost the plans of the Reformer Clara gave him, so Endelman took the measurements from one of Fletcher's Reformers. Endelman agreed to make the Reformer for eight hundred dollars and as he told me recently, "I lost my shirt so for the next few, the price was sixteen hundred dollars."

At first Endelman hesitated about making equipment he knew nothing about, but as a custom furniture maker and meticulous craftsman he enjoyed a challenge, even though this one was odd. So, he accepted more orders for Reformers. Pretty soon, the celebrity waterbed maker was a Pilates Reformer maker. By so doing Endelman unintentionally and unknowingly entered the chain of saviors of Pilates and became its last link.

Endelman, like everyone before him, had no idea that Pilates would become what it is today. He thought he was making a few pieces of unusual equipment with a limited purpose. For those who wanted to open studios, or even teach from their homes, having a source of well-made equipment was essential. Endelman met that requirement. Making exercise equipment for Pilates teachers was a rocky, uncertain enterprise. But the orders kept on coming, much to Endelman's surprise.

In 1980 Endelman discontinued making anything other than Pilates equipment. He moved his family and his shop from the 1,200-square-foot workroom in Northridge, California, to a 1,600-square-foot space in Sacramento. He chose Sacramento because his wife had a job offer paying enough to support the family while he shifted from furniture maker to exercise-equipment maker.

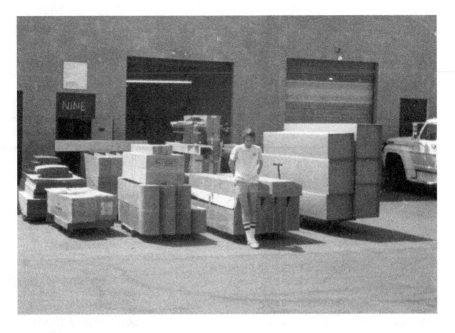

Ken Endelman at his first facility in Sacramento, California, in 1980.

Endelman produced "custom" equipment on demand, meaning he filled orders and personally delivered them, mostly to the Los Angeles area. Ten years later, starting in 1990, the demand allowed him to build equipment on spec, and he took his first regular paycheck. He also hired a truck driver to deliver the equipment, saving him fifteen trips a year. Now, thirty years later, Endelman has the largest share of a robust Pilates equipment industry. He employs over two hundred people in a modern 100,000-square-foot energy-efficient factory, his fourth expansion in Sacramento. And he is out of space again. Endelman's equipment, from the one-at-a-time special-order pieces he made to the semi-mass-produced and varied line of today, is as it was from the beginning: beautiful, durable, and the Rolls-Royce of the equipment industry. The availability of reasonably priced, reliable equipment was vital for the growth of Pilates, but Endelman's most crucial role in perpetuating Joe's legacy was still to come.

As Pilates grew, it attracted attention in the small world of exercise instruction. Among those drawn to it was a New York personal trainer named Sean Gallagher. Gallagher worked in a gym on the

East Side of New York named Drago's. Romana Kryzanowska moved to Drago's after the 56th Street studio closed in 1989. She continued to teach Pilates there by appointment. Gallagher, ever on the lookout for how to make a dollar or two, realized the appeal of Pilates and through Kryzanowska saw an opportunity to make easy money. What if only he controlled the name Pilates? Romana must have told him that she was the anointed heiress of Joseph Pilates, and that she taught the only true Pilates. Whether the ownership idea originated with Gallagher or with Kryzanowska we will never know. My bet would be that it was Gallagher's idea because Romana did not think in terms of legal ownership or monopolies and Gallagher did. Kryzanowska knew where to get exclusive rights to the name cheap—from Wei-Tai Hom, her former intern whom she had taught at 56th Street and who had acquired the lease, fixtures, all the Pilates equipment, and the miscellaneous assets when Aris Isotoner had cut its losses. Shortly thereafter, Gallagher purchased, from Hom, all the assets that Isotoner had acquired from the original Pilates investor group many years earlier. Among the assets was a service trademark for Pilates as a proprietary system of exercise, which Aris Isotoner had registered with the United States Patent Office. Gallagher went a step further and immediately registered Pilates as a trademark for equipment, falsely stating on his application that he sold Pilates equipment in commerce.

Gallagher's action revealed his plan. He didn't use the acquired assets to start or augment a Pilates studio, and he didn't make or sell Pilates equipment. All he did was to try to force people using the name Pilates to pay him for the privilege.

It wasn't long before Gallagher put his plan to capitalize on the purchase of the Pilates name into action. Licensing others, who had to use the name to describe what they did or made, had to be easier than teaching Pilates. That was particularly true for Gallagher, who was not qualified to teach and probably couldn't hammer a nail straight, much less manufacture complicated exercise equipment. First, he had to tell everyone using the name Pilates that he owned it, and their use infringed on his ownership. He elected to initiate this process not with a friendly letter but with a notice from a lawyer.

Gallagher's New York law firm sent a slew of truculent cease-and-desist letters to everyone he could identify who was using the name Pilates. The letter gave the users the option to license the name by paying a royalty and conforming to vague standards, or to stop using the name to identify what they did or made. He threatened to sue if the recipient refused a license, and he would seek damages for the user's past, although unknowing, infringement. Once the letters were out, Gallagher sat back, expecting urgent pleas for permission to use the name, which he was prepared to grant for a limited term in exchange for a fixed annual fee and his right of oversight. His attorneys had prepared a license agreement that Sean intended to offer on a take-it-or-leave-it basis, much as Microsoft does when it lets you buy Word or any of its products.

None of the recipients, longtime users of the name, had any idea who this guy Gallagher was or any understanding of how anyone could own Joe and Clara's name. There were about two hundred Pilates teachers in 1990, almost all working from their homes or small studios. They were panicked, as none could afford tribute to Gallagher for use of a name identifying what they had learned and now taught. Among the recipients of the letters were several enterprises so closely identified with the name that they could not abandon its use. In that group were Fletcher's Studio and Endelman's manufacturing business.

Fletcher, who like several other teachers had learned from Joe, and Endelman, who manufactured equipment starting with a model Reformer made from plans provided by Clara, could not accept that the name could be taken from them. No one, with rare exception, was amenable to paying for continued use of the Pilates name. That its reputed owner was an unknown person in New York, who didn't know or teach the work, made the demand that much more offensive. Fletcher, who initially did his best to avoid Gallagher's sting, and in any case had for years used alternate names, was incensed. He refused to acknowledge that someone owned the word Pilates, even if he didn't need to use it. He owed loyalty to Joe and Clara's memory, and was ready, willing, and able to resist Gallagher's attempt to exploit what he and others were convinced was a bogus trademark registration.

How ridiculous of Gallagher to ask Fletcher to pay for something that Fletcher had revived from near extinction. Adding a requirement that Fletcher conform to someone else's interpretation of Pilates to preserve the "purity" of the name was beyond ludicrous; it was an outrage. After all, Fletcher had been approved and legally licensed in writing by Clara! And to the extent that Gallagher's purchase had any value at all, the value was created mostly by Fletcher.

Challenging Fletcher was a costly mistake, but not his worst. Gallagher's most damaging misjudgment was pissing off Endelman, who, in addition to being tough, street smart, and principled, was a brilliant organizer and eager to lead and financially support whatever it took to deny Gallagher's claim. Gallagher's increasing demands were unacceptable. Greed causes misjudgments, I suppose. This error awakened and released the caged lion in Endelman, perhaps channeling Joe. The lion was now out on the streets and very dangerous.

Shortly after Sean mailed the cease-and-desist letters, I received a call at my law office in Telluride, where I had been living since 1990, from Joan Breitbart, whom I had known vaguely as a fellow client at the 56th Street studio back in the 1970s. Joan Breitbart left New York and had started an organization in Santa Fe, New Mexico, called the Institute for Pilates Method, which was one of a few outposts promoting the revival of Pilates. Breitbart received a cease-and-desist letter and was following the flow of similar letters to others. She had recalled from her New York days my involvement with Joe and Clara and tracked me down. Joan told me about Sean Gallagher's threats and Romana's complicity. Then Joan got right to the point: "Can this guy in New York, Sean Gallagher, stop everyone from using the name Pilates?"

I said, "No, he can't." I went on to explain what I knew about Joe. "Joe's vision was to have everyone do Contrology and neither Joe nor Clara cared about using their name. Joe had not tried to protect the name." I also told Joan what I knew about trademark law. Trademarks can't exist in a vacuum; they identify a product or service from a specific source. That connection protects the consumer (he or she knows what they are getting), and it protects the brand owner (no one else can poach the name). A trademark not connected to a business is invalid. And since Sean didn't seem to be using what he purchased to start a new Pilates studio, that alone would probably invalidate the mark. Joan asked me to call Ken Endelman.

When I spoke with Endelman, he had the same question as Joan Breitbart, and he got the same answer.

Ken filled me in on what had already taken place in his relationship with Gallagher. When Ken got his cease-and-desist letter, he immediately realized that as the leading manufacturer of Pilates equipment, he had to negotiate a license or defend a lawsuit. Either would be costly. Only by defying Gallagher could he eliminate the threat to everyone. If he couldn't make a deal covering everyone who needed to use the name, and Gallagher sued and won, Endelman and his customers would be out of business, and he would be back to making waterbeds.

Endelman told me he had contacted Sean in response to the letter. Back-and-forth negotiations ensued, and every time Endelman thought he had a deal, Gallagher either increased the licensing fee or changed the terms. More negotiations followed. Ken Endelman finally gave up negotiating. He was convinced Gallagher could not be dealt with and had to be resisted.

With negotiations at a stalemate, Ken began his journey to the federal district court. He had no experience with litigation, no idea of how long it would take or how inconvenient it would be or what it would cost, but he was determined to see it through. His business depended upon it, and his integrity demanded it. Ken asked whether he could have my help. I gladly volunteered to be available for whatever he needed, including just talking things over. I was not his lawyer and had no interest in getting involved as a lawyer in this controversy. But I did want to help. I knew I would be a witness.

Both Endelman and Gallagher were fated to collide. Gallagher, to enjoy the income from his purchase, had to collect a significant royalty from Ken Endelman's manufacturing company, Balanced Body. Gallagher thought Endelman would be an easy mark: Balanced Body had to continue to use the Pilates name. Believing there to be no alternative, as Gallagher did, was his next mistake. Gallagher didn't know

Endelman, and he didn't know the limits of his own assumed leverage. Endelman, too, had his blind spot: he didn't know the extent of Gallagher's greed nor did he know he was dealing with a dangerously unreasonable person—a fool.

After our first telephone conversation, Ken would phone me from time to time to bring me up to date and vent a bit about the frustration he was experiencing with Gallagher. Ken told me that he had gone back and forth with Gallagher for six months with Gallagher getting more and more belligerent and truculent. Endelman terminated negotiations and continued to use the name. Gallagher finally pulled the trigger and served Endelman with legal papers during Endelman's Christmas Eve family dinner, 1995. Gallagher not only picked the wrong person to sue, he most definitely picked the wrong time to play silly games by serving Endelman on Christmas Eve.

Endelman is a very patient and reasonable person. He is also a very good businessman, principled, and proof that integrity and good business are compatible.

I learned from Ken during the time before the lawsuit started that Ken had spoken to many lawyers, and even people who knew Gallagher, and he learned that Gallagher was all sizzle but no steak. Endelman had support from many equipment customers who told him about their cease-and-desist letters. Ken told me he felt responsible not only for his business but also the businesses of his customers, without whom he would have no business. Plus, he liked his customers on a personal level, and his outrage at Gallagher's manipulation left him with no choice but to go all in.

Endelman organized the resistance. He formed not-for-profit companies using the name Pilates. He established a mailing list of all the Pilates teachers he could identify, totaling almost two hundred. And he coordinated a defense by engaging expert attorneys.

Over the course of our conversations, I told Ken that Joe wanted everyone to do his exercises and never objected to anyone using his name to describe the exercise program. And while I knew of an ancient patent, I did not believe Joe had ever applied for a trademark. I couldn't imagine that there was any intellectual property connected with the name after the 56th Street studio closed its doors. I also confirmed that neither Joe nor Clara extracted a royalty or license fee from the studio at Bendel's, Carola Trier's, or Eve Gentry's studio. Clara did receive a monthly payment from Fletcher, but not for the use of the name. I gave Endelman my assurance that I would testify and cooperate in extricating the name from Gallagher's pernicious grasp, not only to help everyone involved with the rebirth of Pilates, but because of my attachment to Joe and Clara. Who was this guy thinking he could use the Pilates name against what they had worked their entire lives to establish: popularization of their exercise program?

I knew Gallagher's claim was bogus as a legal matter and wrong as an ethical matter. As a longtime aficionado of Contrology, I selfishly wanted to have it available in as many places as possible. I didn't like monopolies as a general matter and certainly couldn't imagine Joe's name being owned by anyone.

I didn't know Gallagher, but after forty years of practicing law, I knew lots of people who made a living from buying a name, or a mining claim or an easement, not to use it, but to force someone who needed the name, or a right-of-way, etc., to pay top dollar as ransom. This was not Romana; hers had to be a different story. She baffled me. I knew she wanted to be seen as the Queen of Pilates, but what did she expect to gain by helping Gallagher extract royalties? Didn't she realize that what he was doing was injurious to her kingdom? Didn't she have sufficient respect for Joe and Clara that she would understand how opposed to Gallagher they would be? Maybe I underestimated Gallagher's power of persuasion.

What I did know was that allowing Romana, or anyone as a matter of fact, to be able to dictate to everyone else what was or was not Pilates would kill the resurgence of Pilates. That of course would end Gallagher's royalty stream. It amazed me that neither Romana nor Gallagher saw this.

I decided to try to talk her out of this folly. If she could be turned away from Sean, his endeavor would be stopped. He had no business without her. His cease-and-desist letters would be treated like a prank.

When I called Romana, after many years of no contact, I could tell from her curt, dismissive voice she knew what I was about. She listened as I tried to get her on board with the new, revitalized Pilates movement. But I wasn't talking to a sensible person. I was talking to a diva, the self-anointed successor to Joseph Pilates . . . she had become the mythical person I created for her many years before. My bad, I suppose. She had once been my friend, my Pilates teacher, my kids' ballet teacher, my business partner. She hung up on me.

Like Ken, I got ready for the bitter battle ahead.

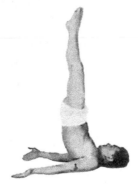

CHAPTER 8

Joe's Legacy on the Scales of Justice

It was a typical New York City June day in 2000—warm, muggy—when the bailiff called the attendees to order in the United States District Court for the Southern District of New York, in the case identified as: Pilates, Inc. versus Current Concepts, Inc. and Kenneth Endelman. It had taken over four years for this case to reach the trial stage. And neither party had caused an unusual delay.

The old-style courtroom was housed in an imposing Classic Revival building at the southern tip of Manhattan. It was a stone's throw from my great-grandfather's once successful clothing store on the edge of Chinatown, long since out of business. I knew the United States courthouse and Chinatown well. Forty years of practicing law taught me two things about litigation: it was slow, and it was unpredictable. Justice was elusive—and expensive.

As I trudged up these steps for the umpteenth time in my career as a litigator, but this time as a witness, I started to think of the irony of this lawsuit. Joe had spent his life hiding from the government, and now his dream for his life's work would be enabled or destroyed by the government he avoided.

The trial that was soon to start was not the first clash in court between Endelman and Gallagher. Sean did not get the response he either expected or hoped for from his original cease-and-desist letters and knew he would have to turn his threat into action. In 1998 he sued one little studio as an example of his determination and power. As his first victim, and the example to frighten everyone else into quick submission, he picked Deborah Lessen, a Pilates teacher in New York, with a small studio, who had been trained by a student of Joe's. Because of her location, her credentials, and her reputation, she was a competitor of Romana's.

Lessen had started the Greene Street Studio in 1983. She had taught Pilates for ten years. She identified what she did and her studio as Pilates. One evening, sitting in her living room, she was served with papers summoning her to federal court. Sean Gallagher was seeking a court order to stop Lessen from using Pilates to describe what she taught. He also wanted "damages" for Lessen's past use of the name. Gallagher, in his usual rude way, hadn't called her or made any contact; he just sued her. The process server arrived, according to Lessen, "like a meteorite in my living room." Lessen retained Lawrence Stanley to defend her. Smart choice. Stanley knew about Pilates and knew intellectual-property law. His response: "This is a hoax; Gallagher has no rights; you must fight back."

And fight back she did. To support her legal costs, she contacted other Pilates teachers around the country, all potential infringers, who generously chipped in. Lessen even had a fundraiser in New York. But what kept her going was Ken Endelman's support. He pulled the heavy financial oar. Her case was subsequently consolidated into the Endelman case.

Ken Endelman retained Gordon Troy, a very competent, down-to-earth Vermont attorney. Ken, along with several studio owners, formed a not-for-profit charitable corporation named Joseph H. Pilates Foundation to, among other things, act as a shield against Gallagher. Like the bull charging the red cape, Gallagher sued the foundation, which elected to conserve litigation funds and settled. Sean Gallagher's scorched-earth strategy scored a victory, which convinced Gallagher he could outlast Endelman, even with a flimsy claim.

Ken's tactic was a mistake, but fortunately not serious. Despite the momentary legal loss, Ken continued to use Pilates to describe his products. Sean started suit against Ken personally and Ken's company. Ken denied Sean's claim of ownership and moved to invalidate the trademarks. This was the mother lawsuit, the lawsuit about to be tried upstairs in this very imposing courthouse.

Shortly after Gallagher started the lawsuit, he scored a victory in the pre-trial maneuvers against Ken. Ken had obtained the court's permission to form a class of all those that used the word Pilates. There were several good reasons for Ken to bring all the Pilates people into one lawsuit, including judicial economy. It was a gamble. If it worked, everyone could use the name Pilates. If it failed, no one could use the name. There was psychology involved: the court would see how many businesses used the name. Because Ken requested the class, he was required to pay the considerable expenses of getting everyone on board. When faced with the extraordinary costs of forming a class, Ken and Troy decided not to spend money consolidating all the Pilates people in one lawsuit. Ken and his lawyers reasoned that the class was not necessary; if Ken won the non-class lawsuit, the trademarks would be invalid, and anyone could use the name without fear of Gallagher. If he lost the lawsuit, that would be bad for him and would set a difficult precedent, but it didn't bind anyone else. Ken petitioned the court to undo the class. Gallagher must have been heartened by Ken's change of mind, correctly assuming it was for lack of money. Gallagher saw this as a win because Ken blinked. This boost, combined with the earlier victory shutting down the foundation, must have convinced Sean that just a little more punching, just a little more truculent saber rattling, and Endelman would fold. Gallagher would win the war by a settlement. After all, bullying had worked so far.

When all the posturing and negotiating ended, and the trial started, and resolution one way or the other was a certainty, the reawakening of Pilates and the survival of the growing businesses it had spawned were to be decided by presiding judge Miriam Cedarbaum. The case could not have landed before a better judge. Miriam Cedarbaum, a New Yorker through and through—Brooklyn's Erasmus Hall High School, Barnard College, and Columbia Law School—had been a federal judge for fourteen years. She had yet to make her mark in the specialized law of trademarks. The Pilates case would be the start of it. Subsequently, Judge Cedarbaum became known for her decision in the dispute over ownership of Martha Graham's choreography. (Truly a coincidence that Martha Graham had been a client of Joe's and had sent many a hurt dancer to him, including Ron Fletcher.)

Cedarbaum was smart, disciplined, attentive, and a typical New York Southern District no-nonsense jurist. She was tough on lawyers, but if you wanted justice, you were very fortunate to have Miriam Cedarbaum presiding. If you had an angel on your shoulder, she would see it. Or if the devil was behind you, she would see that too. Miriam Cedarbaum had been around the block, an essential journey for any judge before sitting nearly immobile on the bench. She came to the law, and to the bench, to do justice.

When the bailiff struck the oak gavel on the oak block on the judge's bench, and simultaneously commanded "All rise," the process was underway to determine whether one word, "Pilates," was descriptive of a system of exercise and thus belonged to the public, or whether it was "property" as identifying a specific unique service or the manufacturer of equipment.

Resolving this dispute wasn't simple. It wasn't a matter of common sense. It wasn't a matter of fairness and equity. It was a matter of the creation of private property by law. If Pilates, a person's name, was private property, like Ford, for example, then Ken Endelman conceded he and all the Pilates people were using the name like squatters on a piece of property: they were trespassers on Sean's rights. Was the court going to evict them despite their long use of the name and dependence on it? The law favors the rights of property owners and gives no quarter to those who trespass. A starving person can't go on someone's lawn without permission and pick an apple off the owner's tree.

Stakes were high on the outcome of the case: If the court granted private property rights to Sean, then he could squeeze as much as he wanted from anyone who needed to use "Pilates" to describe what they provided or made. He could deny use of the name and shut them down altogether. He would have a monopoly and he, and those he licensed, could be the only ones to claim they provided Pilates. It was all or nothing for each party: there was no middle ground. To add to the tension, the judge's decision was final as a practical matter. The loser could appeal. But there was only a slim chance of overturning a careful and smart judge. Judge Cedarbaum rarely made an error serious enough to have her decision reversed. And the big part of her job in this case was fact-finding. There was no jury to find the facts. Once the judge found the "facts," they were rarely challenged.

Facing the judge, sitting at the table on the right, were the plaintiff, Sean Gallagher, and his attorneys. Ken Endelman and his lawyers sat at the table on the left. For me, sitting behind the bar as a spectator, a victory for Sean wouldn't change my life. It would be an emotional blow. I would be upset if Joe's name could be commercialized by Gallagher, a person he would despise, and his exercise program controlled by Romana, who as a self-anointed disciple was an imposter, someone he treated for an injury and never certified to teach. And, on another level, seeing the law, to which I had devoted my life, result in what I perceived as a massive injustice would be disheartening. Sitting with me were approximately fifty spectators—almost the same number of people who did Contrology in 1967, the year Joe died. A few were aligned with Gallagher; most were Pilates teachers whose livelihoods were at stake and threatened.

Judge Cedarbaum, sitting high on the bench, had to ignore everything outside the facts as they were presented to her. Her task was to sift through the evidence and establish her version of the facts. The law, as Judge Cedarbaum understood it, would then be applied to the facts as she found them. Theoretically, she had to be indifferent to the consequences on the lives of those facing her. Was justice, with all the subjectivity about the facts and the judge's interpretation, really blind? How well Judge Cedarbaum did her job was strictly a personal matter. She answered to no one: she was appointed for life.

As soon as the trial started, it was obvious that Judge Cedarbaum had no idea about Pilates. She did not know what Pilates looked like in its natural habitat—the studio. So the ever-cooperative plaintiff's attorney, Kenneth Bressler, Esq., whom I had opposed years ago in another case, suggested to the judge that she come to Romana's studio and see for herself what Pilates was all about. Endelman's attorneys, Robert Fogelnest and Gordon Troy, preferred a neutral site but had no valid reason to dispute this selection. After all, they did not want to appear to be defensive.

The next court day would start in the studio where Sean and Romana worked: Drago's "the Gym" on New York's posh East Side, down a block or two from Tiffany's, Bergdorf Goodman, and Henri Bendel. Transporting the court so the judge could see Pilates in action required a minibus for the court personnel: the judge, her clerk, the court stenographer, the bailiff, and security. The parties to the lawsuit and their legal teams were to arrive on their own. Once there, they all crowded into a small studio where Romana had set up a Reformer and engaged one of her young teacher-trainees to act the part of the customer.

Romana was in her element. This was her glory day. She put the student through a "classical" à la Romana routine, making corrections in her gravelly voice. Romana sought to convince the judge the Pilates being demonstrated was the only Pilates—"because it was exactly as Joe Pilates taught it," she said. She neglected to point out that she had adjusted movements and altered positions to conform to her aesthetic as a ballet teacher. She even used ballet terms such as "second position" or "plié" in her instructions. Her customers, at an earlier time when I was one, didn't care what she called anything nor did we mind the adjustments, although Joe would have shivered at the thought that Contrology had been infected with ballet terms.

Things up at Drago's went well for the plaintiff, Gallagher, or so it seemed, as the judge took in the very precise and special choreography that Romana demonstrated. The student obeyed Romana's cues to perfection. Both Romana and the student were beautiful to behold—Pilates as art, Pilates as a precisely choreographed ballet. The demonstration was convincing: this, and only this, was Pilates . . . a precise system developed by and the property of Joseph Pilates, properly transferred through legal documents. Plaintiff's attorney had to be congratulating himself on his strategy of bringing the judge to a viewing at Drago's gym. The scales of justice were tipping his way.

But, as happens all the time on television (though rarely in an actual courtroom), a thunderbolt struck. When Romana's demo of the "true" Pilates was over, and the student was sufficiently worked out and sweating, the judge turned to the young lady and casually asked, seemingly out of personal curiosity, "How was that for you?" (Judge Cedarbaum had a wicked and sometimes off-color sense of humor.)

The student said: "It was great, but very different from the Pilates taught by Kathy Grant, my former teacher."

What? Different from Kathy Grant's Pilates? Who, asked the judge, was Kathy Grant? Troy, Ken's lawyer, gladly supplied the answer. "Kathy was one of only two people certified by Joseph Pilates to teach. She was certified in 1964, after twenty-two hundred hours of apprenticeship to Mr. Pilates. Kathy ran the Pilates studio just up the block in Bendel's with Joe's permission for many years and now she teaches Pilates at New York University in its world-renowned Tisch School of the Arts." Troy added that Kathy Grant would testify as a witness.

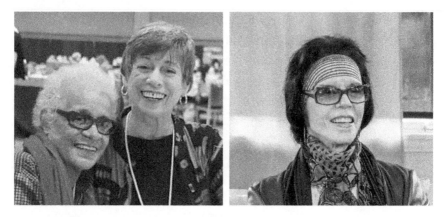

Left: Kathy Grant and Lolita San Miguel, beloved master Pilates teachers taught by Joe. Right: Mary Bowen, another "elder" taught by Joe.

Romana's student had opened a severe crack in Gallagher's case. And as the late poet and songwriter Leonard Cohen pointed out, the crack is what allows the light in. And this little ray of light raised foundational questions: Two different Pilates? From two well-established teachers both connected to Joseph Pilates? The response of the student must have rattled around in the judge's mind. Wasn't plaintiff Gallagher claiming he owned the only one? Here in front of the judge was a student already exposed to two sources, each, according to her, different from the other.

Gallagher's attorney, Ken Bressler, suddenly had to wonder if he had the better case—or even a good case. Clearly there were problems ahead. This judge was sharp. Bressler was a smart lawyer and must have realized he needed more than a demonstration, and a chain of title, to establish the validity and enforceability of a trademark. Had Bressler's client told him the whole story? Time would tell. The demonstration was only a prologue. And the student wasn't under oath. Bressler, after the momentary shock, had to believe he could recover; most of the trial still lay ahead.

Back in the courtroom it came time for Gallagher's side to put on their witnesses, and Romana was called to the stand. She was composed, warmed by her satisfaction with the earlier demonstration. And skilled as a practiced performer. Romana testified that the system of exercise called Pilates had been entrusted to only her by "Uncle Joe," as she referred to him. Romana was emphatic: she taught Pilates exactly as Uncle Joe prescribed. He wanted her to make sure that everyone followed his movements with precision.

Sitting in the courtroom, I knew differently. Romana had last done Contrology under Joe's tutelage in 1944, when she was a teenager. What she did then was not the full routine every client of Joe's did, but a specialized routine designed by Joe for her specific injury at the time. Over twenty years later, in 1972, when she became the manager/principal of the new studio, she had to relearn the routines. John Winters, Joe's former assistant, quickly brought her up to speed. She learned what she had to quickly and accurately.

I reflected on my role in encouraging Romana to believe she was Joe's successor. When I sold her on taking over the studio a long time ago, my suggestion was an appealing fiction. I thought, mistakenly, she understood that. Romana, who was long familiar with playing roles, loved the part so well she inhabited it. At the time I forgave myself for what I thought to be but a white lie because I believed it was harmless pretense: a desperate expedient with no thought that Romana or Pilates would ever be sufficiently important to end up in federal court. It was appropriate for Romana to take on the role of master teacher in the 56th Street Studio, but the notion she was the sole, unchallengeable arbitrator of who could use the word Pilates was unthinkable. I knew Joe would not have anointed her, or anyone else, to this position.

Romana was under friendly questioning by Bressler, Gallagher's attorney. She told her story with all the humility a diva could muster, which wasn't much. Her testimony was all about her role, her importance, and the necessity she arbitrate what was and was not Pilates as Sean's agent. I sat there wondering how anyone, including Romana, could tell if a certain exercise was or was not Pilates? I couldn't tell, and I had spent years with Joe. Joe even changed it for different people or just when he felt like it.

Romana's position was preposterous, and if there was no evidence on what standards were to be applied, I was certain the judge would have a problem with the notion that one person was to be anointed the decider of what was and was not Pilates. I handed a note to Ken for Gordon Troy pointing out this omission and suggesting he avoid this topic. I knew Romana well enough to know she would come up with something if Bressler pressed her for a workable standard. Bressler didn't ask her how she could tell one way or the other, and I breathed a sigh of relief.

Like all good trial lawyers, Gordon Troy, sitting next to Ken, had a finely tuned ear for personality traits that could be exploited. Romana's self-involvement and dramatic flair were hard to miss, and he saw an opportunity to use Romana to bolster Ken's case. This would not be a cross-examination to test her credibility, trip her up with inconsistencies and improbabilities, like those on television. This would be a cross-examination to get her to say too much, to get her to exaggerate.

Troy started his questioning with gentle, respectful leading questions. He encouraged Romana, now sitting impossibly erect, to amplify her role in the world of Pilates. Romana took the bait. She inflated the brilliance of Pilates and how wonderful it was for the mind and body. Romana agreed that dancers warmed up by doing what they referred to as "the Pilates." Troy asked her, "Is the term Pilates when used by dancers used in the way table tennis is called ping-pong?" Romana gave a very clear "Yes."

Bingo! Exactly what Troy wanted. The judge took notes. Troy was on a roll and wanted even more from Romana.

Romana identified many teachers who used the word Pilates to describe their service. She testified they were "scattered" around the United States. She agreed that all the teachers she had trained, and every teacher she knew, identified what they did or taught as Pilates.

Teachers able to provide this important evidence were sitting in the spectator seats facing Romana. And they would be called to testify. But Troy wanted to present this evidence from Sean's key witness first. Romana was an honest and principled person. But even if she were inclined to lie, she couldn't when she knew she would be challenged by Ron Fletcher, Kathy Grant, equipment manufacturer Donald Gratz, orthopedic surgeon Dr. James Garrick, and a handful of established teachers, such as Amy Taylor (Alpers) from Boulder, Colorado, whom

Romana had trained and certified. With only gentle prodding, Romana told the court she had trained hundreds of her students as professional Pilates teachers. She acknowledged there were Pilates teachers whom others had trained. Romana agreed that anyone wanting to do Pilates, say in Omaha, Nebraska, or Denver, Colorado, for example, could find a teacher simply by looking up Pilates in the yellow pages.

Judge Cedarbaum was paying close attention. Romana was an important witness. The judge turned to her and asked: "When people talk about Pilates, whether they do it as well as you, they're not talking about you, they're talking about this method of exercise, correct?"

There it was, the one fact that determined who would win. Pilates was either connected to Romana, and Gallagher would prevail, or it was descriptive of a method of exercise, and Gallagher would lose and his trademarks become worthless. Which would it be? The case hung on Romana's answer.

Romana responded spontaneously: "I hope so."

By that flip but sincere response, Romana conceded that Pilates was considered by the consuming public to refer to a method of exercise. Someone wanting to do Pilates could find it anywhere. They wouldn't think they had to go to Romana or Sean to find it.

By the time Romana stepped down, Gallagher's case was in shambles. Troy turned to Ken and said: "I think we got it." Sean, seemingly still unaware of the legal requirement for a trademark that it identify a particular source, stood and hugged Romana. Hers was a good performance but, seemingly unknown to Sean, a losing one. Apparently, Sean's attorney hadn't questioned Romana before he filed the lawsuit. Too bad Sean and Romana were not advised when they first sought legal representation that their legal claim as owners of Pilates was shaky. Perhaps Sean's lawyers didn't anticipate the evidence. Perhaps Sean and Romana wouldn't listen to their lawyers. It didn't matter anymore. When Romana's testimony was concluded, it was clear that she and Sean were on the wrong side of the evidence. The cease-and-desist letters were bogus, hollow threats, which unfortunately took a great effort to deflate.

Romana, the one person who could have brought everyone together toward establishing minimum standards to become a certified Pilates teacher, had, by supporting Sean Gallagher and insisting on her prominence, cleaved the community into two camps. In her camp, the originalists or classicists, or those claiming that they taught the true Pilates, were those she had personally trained. Even today they are referred to as "Romana people." All the other teachers, many of whom claimed to be classical teachers, even the few teachers still surviving trained by Joe, supported an open Pilates available to anyone who learned and respected it.

Tragically, it was not enough for Romana to be accepted as a great teacher and teacher's teacher, which she was. It was not enough to be credited with and respected for keeping Joe's method and legacy alive. I knew Romana, and I never doubted that her participation in Gallagher's easy-money scheme didn't originate with her. I am sure she fell under Sean's influence. He seduced her, as I had twenty-five years earlier, by appealing to her vanity, her diva gene. It wasn't hard. Her need to be acknowledged as the Keeper of Pilates merged seamlessly with Sean's need to make an easy dollar selling something that was never his.

But even if he sensed his case was unraveling, Sean couldn't call it quits without the strong possibility that the court would make him pay Ken's attorney fees for bringing a frivolous lawsuit. He was having enough trouble paying his own attorney. He pushed onward with true entrepreneurial certainty. After all, the court had not heard Sean's side of the story—a story as he saw it of his innocent purchase of a trademarked name with the purest intention of reviving and preserving Joe's wonderful exercise program. He no doubt thought he could sell this to the judge. He took the witness stand.

Like Romana, Sean proved to be a crucial witness, but for his adversary. To have a valid trademark, Sean needed to connect his purchase of the trademark to an active business. To be private property, trademarks must identify a product or service. Trademarks are much more than names. When questioned by his lawyer, Sean told the story of his purchase from Wei-Tai Hom. Sean testified he bought everything:

the equipment, the customer lists, the goodwill of the customers, and a collection of photographs of Joe and his exercises going back to the 1940s. At this point he had satisfied the "connected to a business" requirement. All he had to do was use the assets as a business, and Wei-Tai's failure could be Sean's success. He had only to stick to this story on cross-examination.

Troy was curious about the acquisition. Was it a business when he purchased it? Sean recounted its recent history, acknowledged it wasn't operating, but stated that all the assets to resume the business were there. Okay, that was passable. Troy pressed on and asked about the purchased assets. What had happened to them? That was easy for Sean: he sold most of the equipment to others, and the goodwill was old, and he hadn't sought to revive the customer base. Troy asked again about the customer lists: Did Sean still have them? Sean didn't have them; he had burned them—along with 80 percent of the archives.

Burned them? Who does that? Shredded, maybe, thrown out, perhaps, but burned? Okay, that sounded fishy, but the legal impact of Sean's testimony was deadly: he admitted he bought all the assets only to get the trademark. The rest were sold or in the fire. There was no business. And the trademark that remained was obtained not by Joe, or even our group, but by Aris Isotoner. Thank you, Sean!

I know I was not alone being astonished as I heard this testimony. Sean and Romana had persisted with a claim their lawyers had to know had no merit. They had threatened to put hard-working Pilates instructors out of business. They had threatened Ken's business. They had incurred huge attorneys' fees, forced others to incur equally large fees, wasted judicial time, and done it with no purpose other than to make a few dollars from someone else's labor.

There was cruel irony involved. Sean lied in court when he testified that he destroyed the archive. We know that now because much of the archive still exists, and Sean sells access to it. During what is termed the "discovery phase" before trial, Ken and Troy had sought to examine the business records and archive Sean had bought. They were looking for evidence of any attempt by Joe to protect his name or the design of his equipment. Troy had served Sean with papers demanding an inspection of these documents. Sean had refused, in a sworn document under oath, on the grounds these documents no longer existed because they had been burned in a fire. Endelman's team didn't believe that story.

Now, on the stand, Sean was trapped in his lie. If he told the truth on the witness stand, he was admitting to perjury back in the earlier discovery stage of the case. If he stuck to his "burned them" story, it was unprovable perjury now, but it crashed his case—no business connection. Troy knew it and Sean knew it. If Gallagher was caught in his previous "burned them" lie by testifying that he still had the customer and business records, his case might have a chance of fulfilling the "business" requirement, but his previous perjury would sink him. The judge might even dismiss it. If Sean stuck to the lie about burning the business records, he would be admitting he had no interest in the business of Pilates, only the name. Sean, by sticking to his lie, handed the judge the evidence to conclude Sean had purchased a trademark separate from a business. Sean owned, in legal jargon, a naked, thus invalid, trademark.

When Troy put on Endelman's defense, the definition of Pilates as a system of exercise was emphasized. Many witnesses, including Endelman and Fletcher, told the court of their history with and use of Pilates. Twenty-four professional teachers testified, some certified by other teachers "scattered around the country," as Romana stated earlier. The exercises and routines taught by professionals varied greatly, depending on the individual teacher's judgment, knowledge, and aesthetics. Each witness confirmed that what they taught was derived from the system developed by Joseph Pilates. Every witness described what they did as Pilates, just as Romana had earlier. Every teacher acknowledged there was no other way to describe what they did, or what their customers did, other than to call it Pilates.

I was called up as a witness for Ken. After recounting the story of my relationship to Joe and Clara, and the history of the business after Joe died, I told the court of Joe's dream to have everyone doing what he then called "Contrology." I testified that Joe and Clara had never sought royalties, and that Joe would be proud that his work was finally receiving acceptance—and it was happening close to the time he had predicted on his deathbed some thirty-three years ago. I testified that the Pilates I did in New York, France, England, Los Angeles, and Telluride were all different but were all Pilates. Neither the judge nor any lawyer asked me how I knew what I was doing was Pilates.

When Judge Cedarbaum issued her opinion many months later, in October 2000, it was clear and devastating. For the winners, it was good reading. For me, all I needed to see was the judge's conclusion, one of many, that "Plaintiff cannot monopolize a method of exercise (or) the generic word used to describe it." So ended Sean Gallagher's ill-fated attempt to capitalize on the work of a man he never knew and a program he didn't understand. Had Gallagher and Romana succeeded, there is good reason to believe that they would have trampled the seedlings that had sprouted steadily since around 1990, from soil essentially dormant since 1967. With the judge's decision, the word "Pilates" became a descriptive term available to anyone. It is now a household word thanks to the tenacity of Ken Endelman, the courage of Ron Fletcher, the genius of Joseph Pilates, and the dedication and passion of the thousands who love the work so much they get up each morning eager to teach it to others.

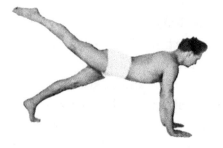

CHAPTER 9

The Origin

Joseph Pilates and his method of exercise had been in the United States for eighty years when I prepared for my first lecture in 2007. Pilates, by then, was taught by thousands, practiced by millions. The name, heard everywhere, had been tested by fire in a federal lawsuit and found to be in the public domain. Yet, surprisingly, no one knew where the exercise program came from other than the mind of Joseph Pilates. What caused him to invent it? No one knew. Joe never revealed or discussed his inspiration. When pushed for an answer, he said, "I know how the human body moves." End of discussion.

The lack of information puzzled me. I, and everyone else, knew Joe had an uncanny sense of the human body. But what inspired him to work out his elaborate program of exercises? Contrology seemed to have popped up right after he arrived in the United States. I sensed, like other aspects of this secretive and mysterious man, Contrology had to be connected to something hidden or embarrassing in Joe's past. I was more than curious, maybe just a shade or two from being obsessed. I started to dig for some evidence, even a strong hint, of where, when, why, and how Joe conceived his exercise program.

I was on a crusade to find the genesis of Contrology. Why had Joe never revealed it? Somewhere in the Joe Pilates story there would be a clue. I started with Joe's history, easily found on the internet. It was very short and suspiciously repetitive. But it didn't have what I was looking for. Joe's footprints were indistinct, and there wasn't a trace about how he came upon Contrology. Everyone who wrote about Joe mimicked the same story in almost the same words. It was a very simple story. Joe left Germany for employment in Great Britain in 1913 or 1914, where he was arrested as a German national and held in an internment camp on the Isle of Man for the duration of World War I. While in camp he organized exercise classes that saved his fellow campers from a cholera epidemic. Upon repatriation to Germany, he was hired by the Hanover police to train their employees. Then in 1926 he left Germany for good, meeting Clara on the boat, falling in love over their mutual fascination with the human body.

I distrusted the story. It was incomplete and much too simplistic. All inquiries led to the same story. Interviews in magazines or newspapers mimicked with suspicious precision the same tightly compressed tale. Nothing in the story touched on the history of Contrology. The trail was cold. I decided to put this quest aside; it was frustrating and not what I had set out to do: writing a book about my time with Joe and a history of modern Pilates. But the questions stayed with me.

Then, in 2014, I came upon a thick, self-published book, published in 2012, entitled *Hubertus Joseph Pilates*, written by a pair of (then) married Spanish Pilates instructors, Javier Pérez Pont and Esperanza Aparicio Romero. Pérez Pont and Aparicio Romero, after several years of total immersion in studying Pilates with Romana to become teachers, had an irresistible urge to find the source of what they were being taught. They knew it was invented by a man named Pilates, but little else. They, too, were troubled by an incomplete history. For seven years they trekked the world trying to find out about

Joe. They followed the geography of Joe's life and even reached far back into his family's ancient German history. Surprise: He was pure German—not Greek, as so many people presumed from his name! And perhaps from the photos and sculptures of him in classic poses. Pérez Pont and Aparicio Romero uncovered documents and checked sources. They noted the absence of documents corroborating Joe's version. They turned their journey into a journal of Joe's life—a very detailed chronology—all in the book. As they fit together the pieces of Joe's life, they checked their findings against his story. Some of the basic facts in Joe's story were either wrong or highly improbable. Some could not be verified. The path they followed was not always congruent even with the sketchy path Joe provided.

I, for one, was amazed by their efforts. It was an act of pure devotion. The chronology developed by Pérez Pont and Aparicio Romero located Joe's every move. But it did not answer the question of where Contrology originated. Nor did it reveal much about Joe himself other than where he had been. It did nothing to dampen my curiosity. Instead, it drove me on. I suspected there was something in Joe's background before his arrival in the United States that helped explain how and why he'd developed Contrology. Joe found Contrology somewhere along the route Pérez Pont and Aparicio Romero had followed. But where, how, and when?

I thought the answer might lie within the contradictions of Joe's story. I began to look in the disconnects and inconsistencies of that story. The first disconnect was the most obvious one: omission by Joe of how he came to develop Contrology. His whole life was Contrology yet there isn't a clue of where it came from. This, to me, was significant. Why? There had to be a reason for his silences and evasions. He had no hesitation about publicly proclaiming the benefits of Contrology in grand terms, but why did he obfuscate its origin?

There certainly was enough information, thanks to Pérez Pont and Aparicio Romero, to allow me to poke about for a coherent story of the man and his method. To the verifiable information, the verifiable misinformation, and the missing information, I added what I knew of Joe and what I knew of Contrology to construct a credible story. I needed to fill in the background to see if I could pinpoint when Contrology popped out.

If my narrative is even close to accurate, it reveals a far more determined and gifted man than Joe's own story portrayed. I came to see that Joe hadn't just invented Contrology; he invented himself.

**

I started with Joe's mysterious decision sometime around December 1913, when he was thirty years old, to suddenly abandon his children and his home in Germany to go to Great Britain. This had to be a pivotal event. Before he left his homeland, Joe lived a typical working-class life. At the time he quit his job, he was a brewer's assistant, a position he had held for twelve years since he was eighteen. Quitting a job and moving on in today's culture of mobility is no big deal. But it was unusual one hundred years ago. Back then people stayed in jobs and marriages. When Joe left town, quit his job, and abandoned his children, it was shocking. There had to be a compelling reason. It wasn't related to Contrology. There was no indication he had any interest in physical training in 1913.

No records indicate the date of Joe's departure from Germany or arrival in Great Britain. He is not listed on any ship's manifest— the only means of overseas travel then available. I arbitrarily use sometime around December 1913 as the departure date because his presence in Germany as late as November 1913 can be verified from documents, and his presence in Great Britain by January 1914 is verifiable. When telling his own story, Joe asserted that the trip to England was for work as either a circus performer or a boxer, depending on which version he was telling at the moment. Neither version can be verified. There are no records from either German circuses or from the circuses then performing in Great Britain establishing that Joe belonged to any troupe. Nor were Pérez Pont and Aparicio Romero able to find verification that Joe boxed in England, though boxing may have been a reason for Joe's decision to move to that country. He did box in Germany before he left. Germany had banned prizefighting—boxing for money—and Joe had been caught and fined for doing so. Another possibility is that he may have traveled, boxed, or performed in a circus under an assumed name, but that would be the only time he ever used an assumed name.

Yet another story of why Joe went to Great Britain exists. This we learn from an interview of August Beinkert conducted around 2010 in New York by Pérez Pont's interview of August John Beinkert, retelling stories told as a memoir by his father, August, middle name unknown. Beinkert Senior's story, as vividly remembered by his son, is interesting and important because Beinkert Sr. was the only witness to Joe's sojourn in Great Britain. According to the story told to August John, the escapade in Great Britain went down as follows.

Beinkert Sr. was a German naval officer disguised as a passenger on a German mine-laying ship, similarly disguised as a passenger ship, that was in the Thames River. Beinkert explained how, in plain sight of the shore and other boats, the captain had surreptitiously laid an underwater mine in the harbor. Later forgetting (or miscalculating) where the mine was located, the ship accidentally bumped into it, quickly refreshing the captain's memory as the ship caught fire and sank. The Brits had to fish Beinkert out of the Thames. Beinkert was immediately taken into custody, and that was the start of a lifelong friendship with Joe. I considered only two possibilities: Joe was on the ship with Beinkert, or Joe was contemporaneously taken into custody on the mainland and they were prisoners together.

Beinkert Sr. recalled a conversation where Joe claimed he had gone to Britain from Germany to take a job as an orderly in a sanatorium. But just like the other two occupations, boxing and the circus, no records have been found of his employment in a sanatorium.

These conflicting and unverifiable employment stories raise doubts that Joe went to Great Britain to work. Joe did not speak English. Changing my inquiry from what pulled Joe to Great Britain, I looked at what may have pushed him out of Germany. Why did he leave?

Joe's timing suggests that his departure was connected to his wife Mary's death in November 1913. Mary died at age thirty-one. Joe went to a neighboring village (one where he didn't live) to file the death certificate, which he had prepared. It is dated November 11, 1913. The death certificate contains a blank space for the cause of her death. Joe had married young. They moved frequently from apartment to apartment, and from one town to another. Joe and Mary had a child, and Joe had adopted Mary's older child from a previous relationship. When Joe took off for Great Britain, he left the two children with Mary's parents. Had Joe intended to leave them there temporarily or permanently? We don't know. Subsequent events—he never saw them again—suggest permanently. And in August 1914, World War I intervened and changed everything. Easy to speculate that grief, guilt, inability to manage the children drove him away from his homeland, but it well could have been something else. Who knows? Even with the facts uncovered by Pérez Pont and Aparicio Romero, this was another dead end. How and why Joe made the trip to Great Britain remains a mystery. And whatever the reason, it does not explain the source of Contrology. But that it is a mystery seems important.

Joe's story of being a civilian in the wrong place (Great Britain) at the wrong time (the outbreak of WWI) doesn't stand up. The first suspicious chink is Joe's lasting friendship with Beinkert from the time of Joe's arrest. Why would a civilian in London be arrested with, even incarcerated with, a German naval officer taken prisoner after mining the Thames River? Beinkert never places Joe on that ship, or even states how he met Joe, but then again, he was never questioned about Joe being on the ship or their first meeting. I suspect from the conversation reported by Pérez Pont and Aparicio Romero that they and Beinkert assumed Joe was on the same ship. Another clue: Beinkert stated that Joe was "captured"—not arrested. Arrest is serious enough; capture implies that Joe was a combatant, adding weight to the supposition that he was on the German mine-laying ship. Subsequent events bear this out. Beinkert and Joe were kept together from the time of their arrest. Whether Joe was a passenger, a stowaway, another German sailor in civilian uniform, or part of the ship's crew doesn't much matter. Accepting that Joe and Beinkert were on the same ship explains why they were arrested at the same time and kept together. It also explains how Joe got to Great Britain without papers and without a trace, as well as the absence of any employment record. Even if Joe was a civilian, his presence on the mine-laying vessel would have caused him to be treated as a prisoner of war, regardless.

An important factor in reconstructing Joe's time as a prisoner was his classification as a prisoner. He claimed to have been a civilian incarcerated because the Brits did not want German nationals running about in England to spy or do sabotage for their homeland. If Joe was a civilian, and apprehended because he was a German, he would have been confined with other German civilians in an internment camp. If Joe was a prisoner of war, then he would have been confined with German military personnel in a POW camp. The conditions of incarceration, even the treatment, would be different for the different groups in different camps.

After Beinkert and Joe were taken into custody, they were sent to the Isle of Man, an island thirty-two miles long and fourteen miles wide in the northern Irish Sea between the coasts of Great Britain and Ireland, and the place of confinement for German nationals, both civilians and prisoners of war. Scant records exist from the Isle of Man. One record shows Joe's confinement there, but for only a four-month stay. Other records show Joe was moved to various other camps on the Isle of Man, some of which were high security. Joe was a prisoner in Great Britain for five years—a significant span in the life of a thirty-year-old.

Beinkert said he was in constant contact with Joe during the four years of the war. This is significant. Beinkert was a German naval officer. That they were kept together indicates that the Brits thought they were the same category of prisoner—German military—and as such, prisoners of war. Beinkert confessed to a serious violation of the rules of war—pretending to be a merchant seaman and mining a harbor full of passenger ships. If Joe was treated like Beinkert, as a POW, his confinement may have been severe and punishing. The Brits could be expected to hate enemy Germans laying mines in their civilian harbors.

I discovered another clue indicating Joe was a prisoner of war and not held as a civilian. Despite his confinement of four-plus years, Joe did not acquire fluency in English. Was it because his incarceration kept him with prisoners of war who only spoke German, rather than with German citizens living in Great Britain who, more than likely, were English speakers?

Joe's version of his background omits any information about his captivity: how he passed the time, what he did, what he ate, or any of the other aspects of life. That Joe never wanted to talk about his years of imprisonment isn't remarkable. Survivors of internment try to put the experience out of their minds. But Joe told one story about his experience on the Isle of Man: the success of his exercise program in protecting his fellow prisoners from a cholera epidemic. That story appears to be made up. There is no mention in the newspapers or the camp's infirmary records of a cholera epidemic on the Isle of Man during Joe's years there. Nor is there any record of Joe promoting or leading an exercise program.

As part of his alleged exercise program, Joe claimed he used the springs on his barracks cot to develop an early version of what would become his signature exercise machine, the Reformer. This story also turns out to be highly improbable. Springs were not used on beds until well after World War I and certainly were not used on barrack cots at the time. The springs eventually used on beds were very short and stiff and would be of no use on an exercise machine like the Reformer, because Reformer springs stretch several feet. Every Reformer Joe built after he arrived in the United States used lengthy, flexible springs, not at all like bedsprings, and to this day Reformers still do.

Another significant piece of evidence is the absence of *any* springs in the drawing Joe included in his patent application for the Reformer, which he filed in the United States in 1926, more than six years after he was released from the Isle of Man where he said he used them. The drawing in the patent application depicts an elevated horizontal platform, on which the user lies. The resistance to movement comes from weights suspended on a rope-and-pulley system. Joe's patented invention was gravity driven with weights, not spring driven. The patent contains a reference to the use of springs as a possibility but without any drawings or description. Gravity was center stage, and the patent application claims the use of gravity as the soul of his

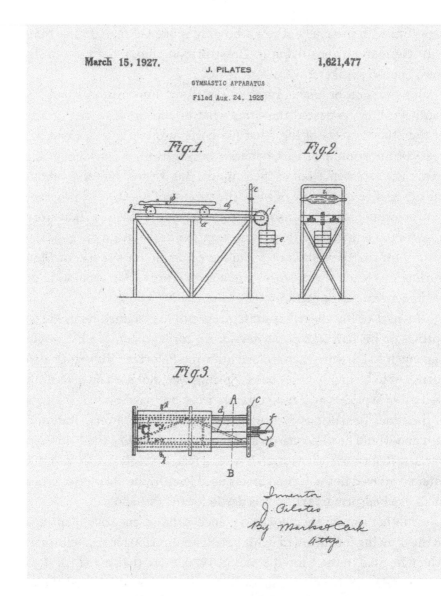

March 15, 1927.

J. PILATES
GYMNASTIC APPARATUS
Filed Aug. 24, 1925

1,621,477

Fig.1.

Fig.2.

Fig.3.

Joe's original Reformer patent. Note the weights at the right in Fig. 1 and the height of the rolling bed. Both the client and the instructor required a ladder, and a high ceiling was required.

invention. To provide enough up-and-down travel for the weights, the platform had to be elevated and the exercise space required a very high ceiling. The person exercising had to climb a ladder to get on the device, and the instructor or therapist had to climb up as well to attend to the client. The gravity-based machine was never built, probably because it was cumbersome and impractical.

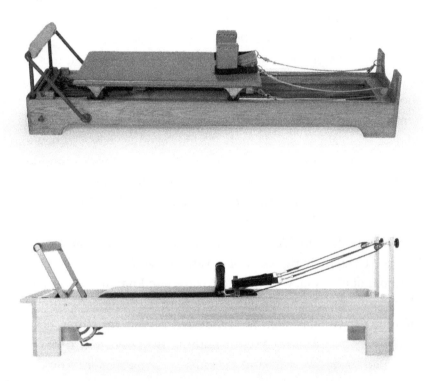

Top: Joe's original Reformer. Note the springs on the left.
Bottom: Balanced Body studio Reformer.

***

Nothing from following Joe's trail helped me to find the source of Contrology. If there had been cholera, and some reference to Joe conducting an exercise program, that would have provided a starting point. And what was this so-called exercise program? Was it Contrology? If so, more layers to peel back. What had Joe left out that might explain how he designed the series of routines we now call Pilates? Why did he invent the cholera story? Perhaps as proof of the benefits of Contrology? Would he have invented it if Contrology did not exist, at least in his mind, at the time? I think not. So I assumed that Joe had a coherent system of exercise on the Isle of Man. Because there is no evidence that Contrology existed before Joe left for Great Britain in 1913, when he was brewer's assistant, I focused on the time while he was on the Isle of Man. I tried to put myself in Joe's situation as a prisoner.

If Joe was a prisoner of war, it's likely he was confined to a small space, like a jail cell or a crowded barrack, with limited freedom to move about. We know Joe loved and needed physical activity—whether as a gymnast, a boxer, a circus performer, or perhaps even a body builder. And he was vain about his body into his eighties, when I knew him. Even late in life, Joe could not sit still: he was always in motion. So what does one do in jail to keep in shape and dispel energy?

I recalled from my career as a lawyer that I had spent a good deal of time handling pro bono prisoners' rights cases. Those cases brought me deep inside prisons to meet with the prisoner committees asserting their rights. If one wants to see buff men, go into the dayroom of a prison, which I had to do when I handled class actions. These guys pass their time either watching television or working out. Joe didn't have television. So, I pictured him at age thirty, stuck in a cell or crowded barrack with nothing to do but kill time. What did he do to stay healthy and sane? He wasn't a reader. Wouldn't he resort to the traditional prisoner activity—exercising his body? The photographs of Joe as a young man more than hint that he was vain. He obviously loved to show off his body and his marvelous physical condition. If his body were a primary focus, he would have to find a way to exercise it.

We can imagine him in his cell, maybe on his cot or the floor, developing and doing what became the mat work of Contrology. Perhaps he studied his body, learning how the muscles worked together or worked in opposition, how to stretch and relax, how to use one set of exercises to stretch or oppose muscles tightened by a previous exercise. And maybe he developed a program for his own use that stretched, tensed, and engaged all his muscles in a fixed order and a rhythm that felt right and was efficient. All this he would have done with no equipment, in hardly any more space than required for a cot.

Joe did not want to talk about his confinement, so if this was where he developed Contrology, it would make sense that he couldn't talk about its origins. Or perhaps he thought it wouldn't look good to connect an exercise program to a prison.

And then there is the mind-body connection that Joe promoted as the soul of Contrology. That, too, could have been a by-product of his confinement. Joe was highly disciplined, even late in his life. In prison he would have been determined to stay fit and stay healthy. Once he got into a routine with an exercise program, the connection between his mental well-being and his physical condition had to have hit him full force. Joe must have noticed his attitude and outlook became positive and his emotional state and physical appearance improved because of the exercises. Joe, like other prisoners, needed exercise as much for his mind as for his body. He would have exercised to save his body and his sanity, just like most of us in or out of prison.

If my hypothesis is correct, then Contrology evolved from a confluence of boredom, Joe's concern for the condition and appearance of his own body, and his extraordinary ability to visualize the mechanics of human movement. He didn't have much to think about or anyone else to worry about in prison, so he most likely spent his time studying how his body worked and how to get the most out of his exercise regime. In that process, he would have acquired an uncanny sense of the connection between muscles, tendons, ligaments, and movements. It's easy to extrapolate from his Isle of Man confinement to his fascination with and study of the movements of caged animals in the New York zoo, a favorite and frequent destination. He was always so excited to watch large animals exercise and stretch, then exercise and stretch again as nature's antidote to confinement.

In his own retelling, Joe claimed that his knowledge of the human body and the principles of Contrology came from reading anatomy books as a child. But it is unlikely that Joe had access to anatomy books in the 1880s or 1890s. Such books were rare in working-class families, and neither of his parents had anything to do with medicine. Even if he had access to them, the childhood reading of anatomy books did not lead him to Contrology: he was forty-three when he identified Contrology as an exercise regime. Furthermore, it's hard to believe that Joe's deep understanding of body movement was derived from the static pictures in anatomy books. During our sessions together, in the thousands of instructions he gave me on what to move, he never once referred to a body part by its anatomical name, as you would expect from a student of anatomy. Joe read your body movement by watching closely, not by referencing it to some ancient anatomical drawings.

If Contrology was conceived while Joe was on the Isle of Man, it remained dormant for some time. Which leads me to the thought that he didn't realize what he had discovered until much later. If his exercises were developed for his prison life, they were personal, and he must have felt that is where they should remain. Perhaps he didn't believe that anyone not as confined as he was would need his exercise program. That belief would have persisted until he came to believe the opposite: everyone needed his program. Perhaps his arrival in New York and the confinement of his life there reawakened his sense of confinement.

Joe's compelling need to make a living upon arrival in New York was, I believe, the event that brought Contrology to life. His system of exercise, grounded in his understanding of the human body's movement, is the one thing he had to sell when he arrived in the United States. And, since he alone knew the real origin of his discovery— likely, his time in prison—he never needed to explain its more unsavory origin.

***

The war ended in November 1918, and Joe returned to Germany in March 1919. He was thirty-five years old, with nothing positive to show for the time between 1913 and 1919. Not that the war interrupted anything significant in his life. When he'd fled Germany five years before, he was just a blue-collar working stiff. He had no job, no career nor any professional skills. On his return to Germany, he faced the same deficits and was five years older. He had decided not to resume work in a brewery, but we know nothing more of the effect of incarceration upon him. During the war Joe had been safely warehoused in Great Britain while his countrymen were being slaughtered, maimed, and humiliated on the battlefield. If Joe left Germany to escape or avoid something, whatever it was may well have been lost, forgotten, or absolved in the chaos of war. He seems to have returned with a clean slate.

As for Germany, it was not a happy place. Its economy was in shambles, its government and political system impotent. The once-proud Germans were humiliated not only by their defeat and the onerous terms of the Treaty of Versailles but by worldwide condemnation for using gas as a deadly weapon. Germany had lost many if not most of its young men, along with its intellectual class, its elitist culture, and its highly esteemed engineering, industrial, and manufacturing economy.

Joe's status as widower did not last long after his return from Great Britain. Curiously, there is no evidence he reunited with the two children he'd abandoned. Instead he found a second wife right away, which must have been easy for a youngish man with his body parts intact—he was a rarity. On October 1, 1919, Joseph Pilates married Elfridge Latteman. They began their domestic life in a small town, Gelsenkirchen, on the western edge of Germany, within miles of Joe's birthplace, bordering Belgium and the Netherlands. Joe had been repatriated for barely six months. Little is known about Elfridge Latteman except she was older than Joe. They soon had a child. From newspapers and advertisements, it appears that Joe was trying to make a living as a boxer and boxing coach. Boxing had been around in Germany for a long time, but it wasn't until the 1920s that it was legal to put on public exhibitions for money. Joe started a boxing school in Gelsenkirchen or an adjacent small town—it is not known precisely where—and he and his pupils put on exhibition matches. The boxing school failed and closed.

The failure of his boxing business once again put Joe's scrappiness and survival instincts to the test. He turned his attention to becoming a sports teacher. The seeds of what Joe might have learned and developed in confinement germinated. And he took it one step further—he invented exercise equipment. On May 4, 1923, Joe applied for a German patent for an exercise device for problem feet, which reduced discomfort and restored function. The device—still sold today as Joe's Toe Gizmo—had a small flexible spring about the size of a cot spring, but not as stiff. Joe had to see commercial possibilities in this device to go to the trouble and expense of obtaining a patent. There is no record that he even marketed it.

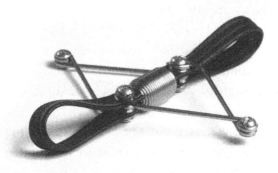

Joe's Toe Gizmo. Note the short spring.

The year 1923, four years after Joe's return, was significant. Joe's brother Fred left Germany in July, intending to settle permanently in Saint Louis, Missouri. In August, Joe separated from Elfridge and moved to the much larger city of Hanover, leaving her and their child behind. There he continued to promote himself as a sports teacher. And in Hanover we see a transformative change: he worked with dancers and dealt with their physical problems. Hanya Holm was one of the dancers who came to him in Hanover. How he made this contact is unknown. Holm was famous in Europe and subsequently repatriated to the United States, where she became much more famous and where she reappeared in Joe's New York life.

Joe booked first-class passage on a steamship from Hanover to New York, departing October 6, 1925. Subsequent events confirm that the trip's purpose was to check out New York as Joe's next move. Once again, what appears to be the impetus for a precipitous and drastic move by the peripatetic Joseph Pilates is unexplained. He may well have been fed up with his life in Germany for many reasons: rampant inflation, political instability, his frustration in business or with his personal life, or something entirely different. The real reason is anyone's guess.

That Joe bought a first-class ticket for his trip to New York is a jarring—but possibly important—detail. The Joe I knew was not someone who sought first-class treatment. And back in the 1920s, there is little indication that he could afford it. But the expensive ticket reputedly provided an unusual advantage: first-class passengers supposedly breezed through entry into the United States—no questions asked. Presumably US customs officials believed that if you could afford first class, you were free from communicable diseases, so you would not be a burden on the state, and according to the same faulty logic, you were not an undesirable nor had a criminal past.

Joe declared that he had eight hundred dollars when he arrived in New York. For a man of Joe's background, that's a great deal of money, especially given the punitive exchange rate of German marks into dollars. Joe may have inflated the stated amount to ease his entry.

Picture Joe's arrival: He bounds down the first-class gangplank to the pier and steps on US soil with his energetic, somewhat bow-legged stride to begin his investigation of New York. He wonders: Is this the place to start all over? Is there some way to earn a living? Do Americans care about exercise? Will they listen to or patronize a German? He asks these questions of himself, as there is no one at the pier to meet him. Even if there were someone there, Joe doesn't speak English, or so he had claimed to the US consulate in Germany when he'd applied for a visa shortly before his departure. If there was a time and a place for Joe to reinvent himself, it had to be upon arrival in New York. He may have known the paperwork he needed to gain entry to the US and had prepared his story long in advance. And he may have anticipated seeking permanent residence in the United States. Here was his golden opportunity to construct a workable story that would enable him to become a resident and then even a naturalized citizen.

The US had not joined the newly founded International Criminal Police Commission (which would later become known as Interpol), and it would be another thirteen years before the US had access to centralized records of international crime. He must have realized that whatever he told the immigration authorities could not be checked but had to be consistent. His past, and anything he wanted to hide, was obscured by the Atlantic Ocean and inaccessible to the US immigration authorities.

Whatever Joe did or found in New York on that first trip must have been to his liking, or at least was an improvement over his situation in Germany. He had to notice the vigor and energy in New York. He had to notice immigrants and refugees from all over the world. No one seemed to care about anyone's history. Germans were treated like everyone else.

***

After two months in New York, Joe returned to Hanover in January 1926. Immediately he prepared to go back to New York, but the return was on a one-way ticket. He needed a new US visa. He needed other documents from his birthplace, so he had his estranged wife, Elfridge, obtain and bring them to him in Hanover. By April 1926, he had all the necessary papers to return and gain entry to the United States. He left Elfridge and their child behind—nothing new. Convincing Elfridge to bring his papers and probably some money to Hanover must have been masterful.

He boarded the SS *Westphalia*; this time he traveled second class. Perhaps now that he knew the immigration procedures, he saw no real advantage to entering the US with a first-class ticket. Or maybe he didn't have the money. Or, on further speculation, he may have had a companion whose ticket he also had to buy.

Sometime before docking in New York, Joe claimed to have met Clara Zuener on the *Westphalia*. A more likely story is that they established a relationship in Hanover and fled together to the United States to start life over. Joe was still married. Either way, Clara Zuener was a second-class passenger aboard the SS *Westphalia*. Clara, who stated her occupation as a domestic servant on her customs declaration, left Germany for unstated reasons. She had five dollars with her; Joe claimed five hundred dollars this time. According to Joe's story, he and Clara were both passionate about studying movement of the human body and what they could do to make a living by using their knowledge to improve people's lives. And because of that shared bond, they'd fallen in love on the voyage over.

Yet much is left out. While crossing the North Atlantic and inhaling the crisp air from melting icebergs, did Joe tell Clara he had now abandoned his second wife, two children by different marriages, and one stepchild? While holding hands watching the sunset from the port deck, or the Northern Lights from the starboard side, did Joe explain that he was coming to the US because his prospects, uncertain though they may be in the US, were far better than anything he could imagine in Germany? Maybe he told her that the chaos in Germany scared him, or that the prospect of military conscription was not for him. Maybe he talked about a plan to save the world through Contrology and the exploitation of his invention. No one will ever know, but whatever was said or left unsaid, a bond was formed that would last their lifetimes.

Whether they knew each other beforehand or they met on the voyage over, they were united in wanting to shed their old lives. When questioned on Ellis Island, Joe had good reason to recast his history, downplaying or perhaps omitting the story of his confinement on the Isle of Man, his illegal entry into Great Britain—even perhaps his reasons for leaving Germany. After all, Joe was seeking admission to the United States less than ten years after the war ended. It would be foolish to tell the US immigration authorities he was in the German navy, mining British waters, if that was indeed true. Or that he was a stowaway and picked a boat that he thought was a passenger liner but turned out to be a minelayer. Bad choice. Perhaps he felt he needed to conceal his history from Clara, who was likely standing right next to him as they entered the country. Either way, no one in 1926 could contradict his version of events. Nearly a hundred years later, we are still in the dark.

I can see Joe and Clara on the pier in New York in 1926, where they sloughed off their pasts like the shells of armor crabs. They descend the gangplank in New York Harbor, presumably arm in arm, the way Joe always walked with me forty years later. From their first encounter with authority they told their story: cryptic biographies that provided just enough information to explain their backgrounds and presence in New York, but not so much to raise questions about their character or cause black marks on the immigration forms. That Joe likely created a story for Ellis Island probably does not differentiate him from a great percentage of the people immigrating to the US. But why did he stick to that story for the rest of his life?

From the moment Joe and Clara arrived on Ellis Island, their lives started anew. New York had to become home. Joe's gym opened in 1927 on 939 Eighth Avenue, where it remained until two years after his death—forty-two years all told. Joe survived on his ability as a physical therapist, the exercise program he named Contrology, and his contacts in the dance world. The dance celebrity Hanya Holm reconnected with Joe in New York and brought him into the dance world, perhaps on a visit before she settled in New York in 1931. Holm became a star in the United States and is credited with being one of the founding pillars of modern dance. Joe became the go-to guy for dancers needing physical therapy. And dancers hurt themselves constantly.

If Joe immigrated to the United States to surgically amputate his past, he succeeded brilliantly. To the extent there was anything questionable in his history, it was, and remains, well concealed. Elfridge divorced him in 1930, in Germany. He was naturalized as a US citizen in 1935. During the 1940s through the 1950s, he was renowned as the only person who could fix broken dancers. His clients included such luminaries as George Balanchine and Martha Graham. In fact, Hanya Holm and Joe developed the warm-up exercises used to this day by many prominent dance companies. In the New York world of dance, Joe became a celebrity, comparable to today's plastic surgeons for movie stars. He also worked with many famous opera singers to improve their breath control.

By the time I met Joe, in 1963, the glory days were rapidly fading. Joe and Clara were two old people hanging on to a diminishing business. Contrology was hardly known outside the dance world, and Joe no longer had the drive to spread its message. Despite his nearly extinct business and failed mission, Joe remained certain that Contrology was a sure means to health and happiness, but that it would take another forty years for the world to awaken to his discovery.

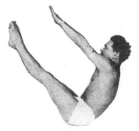

CHAPTER 10

The Deep Attraction

Contrology/Pilates survived in a state of limbo for thirty some years after Joe's death awaiting a spark. Those who did it before Joe died continued to do it. Those few who taught it before Joe died continued to teach it. Why? Why had this small cadre of Contrology loyalists continued to come to a gym that was basically unsupervised after Joe's death back in the late 1960s? Why had anyone volunteered to keep the doors open? Why did people invest money and time in a hopeless venture in the 1970s? Why did Romana become so passionate about it? Why had Joe's former assistants kept at it? Obviously, it wasn't Joe. He was long gone. Suddenly millions started doing it. Why? There has to be something about Contrology that became indispensable first to a small group and eventually to a huge population. And it wasn't merely exercise. There were alternatives. What caused Ken Endelman to bet the ranch—specifically risk his carefully developed business—on a lawsuit against a determined adversary? Why was the name so valuable to Sean Gallagher? Ron Fletcher didn't have to get involved: he had a non-infringing name. But he did. Why?

I never gave a thought to the attraction behind Contrology until one day, after I started this book and was telling a friend about the history of Pilates. My friend asked why I and others felt that it was vital to keep it going after Joe's death. "After all, it is just calisthenics in a different package," he quipped.

I scratched my head and said, "It does seem like a weird form of calisthenics, but it isn't. There is something different that makes you want to continue doing it. You get hooked, but what that something is I really don't know. There is something to Pilates, like there is to yoga, that draws huge numbers of people to it. Pilates differs from all other calisthenic exercise, but I can't explain what that is, although I feel it."

My friend said if I was going to write a book about it, I'd better try to figure it out. I didn't know where to start. I tried to do self-analysis on my reasons for sticking with it for so many years. It was easy to think it was the charisma of Joe. That made no sense for all the others who had stuck with it. That made no sense for the popularity it was enjoying. I asked teachers what attracted them. Why did they want to teach it? They scratched their heads. Most of the answers were that they loved doing it and thought it would be fun to dig deeper and learn to teach. As for their clients, they thought they became regulars because they felt better, but mainly because they "just like it." That, of course, was the question, not the answer. I decided to back-burner trying to get to the bottom of the attraction of Pilates until I had a good part of the book drafted, and maybe it would pop out. And it did.

In 2008 my wife and I checked into a health-oriented, upscale spa in Tucson, Arizona, for a break from our high-altitude life in Telluride, Colorado, where I practiced law and was the mayor. Along with baths, massages of every kind, special diets, and a vegetable juice bar, the spa had many exercise classes, among them a Pilates program. The Pilates studio was in its own space with a separate staff. It was an "extra" or "supplement" requiring a separate fee—something Joe would not have liked. But he wouldn't have liked all the other exercise programs either. I popped into the slick Pilates facility and asked if I could use one of their Reformers after hours, when they had no customers. I told the manager—he had his name and position embroidered on his polo shirt—I knew the Reformer routine and had been doing it for years, but nothing about my personal connection to Joe.

The manager got in a huff and said there was an inviolate requirement that everyone, even experienced Pilates students, even certified teachers, take two private lessons at one hundred dollars each with him or another instructor to be eligible to join a Reformer class at thirty-five dollars a session. Or I could stick with private lessons. He was sorry, but no one could use the Reformer unattended by a "professional," no matter how experienced.

"Insurance," he mumbled.

Hmm, I thought, that is how they stay in business without a local clientele—$340 for six days of Pilates, then tips and taxes, all on top of the daily spa fees. Understandable: teachers need to earn a living, and studio owners just scrape by. But even if I were comfortable with the cost, this was not for me. I didn't like the guy. No need to spend my vacation time starting up with him or an unknown instructor for a one- or two-night stand. I passed.

Late that afternoon I walked by the Pilates studio and noticed no one was inside. The impressive glass double door was unlocked, and the lights were off. Looking all around to make sure I wasn't seen, I walked in. I inspected the Reformer; many studios lock up the spring mechanism to prevent unauthorized use. But all its parts were there. I removed my sneakers and socks (Pilates is best done barefoot), adjusted the springs, and lay down on it. My body slipped into a Reformer routine, and I moved through the basics at a comfortable pace. I was feeling great, not only from the exercise, not only from the pleasure of being alone in the studio, but also because I was being naughty and getting away with it.

I was about halfway through my routine when I noticed a young woman, dressed in skintight exercise clothes, standing in a doorway some ten feet away, watching me. I kept going, accustomed as I was to people in the gym. Moments later she walked over and asked in an authoritarian voice, which didn't fit her teen-like appearance or her flashy athletic outfit, "Who are you and what are you doing here?"

"I'm a guest at the spa, and I am doing a Reformer routine."

"Who said you could use the Reformer? How do you know what to do?"

I told her that no one had said I could use the Reformer—totally true as far as it went. I'd learned the routine and how to do it by myself, from Joseph Pilates.

My observer softened noticeably. She dropped her shoulders, her face relaxed, and she walked back her bossy greeting. She introduced herself with pride, awe, and collegiality as a fellow Pilates instructor, certified by Romana Kryzanowska. She taught part-time at the spa. Despite the evident warmth, she restated what the manager said, this time without the bossy tone: "No outsiders, not even an outside instructor, are permitted to do the routine by themselves."

I confessed that I was not an instructor but only one of Mr. Pilates many students, and I appreciated the rule against outsiders but saw no harm in using the Reformer.

Her curiosity, maybe even amazement that an ordinary person could do a Reformer routine by himself, or that she was in the presence of someone who had learned directly from Joseph Pilates, overpowered her sense of responsibility. "Would it be okay to watch how a student of Mr. Pilates does the routine?"

"Sure." She sat on the adjacent Reformer. I told her not to mention my use of the equipment to anyone because we would both get in trouble. With that we bonded as fellow scofflaws. I continued my routine until it was finished. She thanked me and said she was impressed. Being careful, we left separately. Cheating is risky.

Self-sufficiency was the goal of doing Contrology in Joe's day. It was not only a necessity from Joe's perspective—he couldn't be everywhere—but essential from the client's perspective. Private lessons didn't exist. Joe ran what is today called an "open gym." You came when it suited you. There was something wonderful about that: Everyone was there voluntarily. No one was keeping an appointment. The con: Too few instructors during rush hours (an hour midday and an hour around six p.m.), and too few customers during the slack hours. Joe tried to cover the busy times by scheduling assistants, but only very few were available. Attracting anyone's attention in a crowded gym was difficult. There were times when all Reformers were in use, and the newly arrived client had to start on the mat or other equipment with one eye peeled so he or she could jump on a Reformer when one was vacated. Occasionally, a client would walk in, look around the packed room, make a quick appraisal of where he or she might be in line, and then leave. There was always later or the next day. Standing around and watching were not allowed, and there was no place to sit even if watching had been permitted. Clients arrived, changed, got to work, showered, dressed, and left. During crowded times, finding a place to start took some imagination. Receiving anything more than brief attention, no matter who you were, was not expected. The gym was a small place. Eight people crowded it. Only two people could fit in the locker room at any time, and they had to like each other. Until the client could do the work independently, he or she had to come at a slack time. Hence my regular early morning sessions with Joe in a nearly empty gym with no distractions. He knew that learning the routines was challenging, a slow process, and a struggle, even for dancers, although less so for them. He promised if I could learn to control my body, I could control my life.

Joseph Pilates's gym resembled the fancy Tucson spa only insofar as the name Pilates was on the door. Even the doors were different: Joe's old-fashioned; Tucson's sleek and modern. Once inside, the differences were equally striking. In Joe's gym, talk was forbidden. You couldn't even say hello to anyone—for me that included my parents. You could get away with a head nod or a hand wave. There was no ambient music. Cell phones, headphones, and earbuds were years in the future. Everyone seemed to get along fine without these distractions. There was no reception desk, nor any phone in the gym. Lighting was dim. People moved quietly, and everyone avoided grunting or making any other noise while exercising. Perfume and cologne were prohibited. In an era when many smoked, smoking was forbidden. Everyone arrived in street clothes and changed into a basic workout uniform: women in black or white leotards; men in black shorts, no shirts. Nothing fancier was allowed. No one brought water or could take a break from the routine, even for water. When the gym was jumping, there was a very pleasant hum from the motion of the apparatus sliding back and forth on well-oiled tracks. During the slack time, all you heard were the street noises from Eighth Avenue. The smell, like that of a gym during a high school basketball game, told everyone this was physical work.

It is a rare contemporary studio that imposes the Teutonic discipline of Joe's gym; Pilates is now social. Instructors and their clients, whether in private lessons or in classes, talk to one another. And clients talk to each other before, during, and after classes. Sometimes the conversation is related to exercising: injuries, soreness, medical adventures. More often the chatter is unrelated: recipes, clothes, hair and nails, families, romances, vacations, movies, books, and gossip.

To this day, conversation while exercising disturbs me. It breaks concentration. Background music, prevalent in contemporary studios, along with bright lighting, bothers me as well. I enjoyed the feeling of aloneness in Joe's gym, even when it was busy. I worked better without distraction. There is no dress code anymore and the various outfits, including colorful tights, special shoes, headbands, socks, even workout gloves, catch the eye—as they are meant to do. Not so the boring but soothing dress code of Joe's day.

Today's studios are well designed, nicely lit, chic, with beautiful equipment that is sometimes upholstered in striking colors. Yet the basic exercises and all the equipment are little changed from Joe's times. People come by appointment, and in the larger studios there could be several classes and a private lesson going on at the same time. The energy in modern studios has its own appeal. These studios seem to need a buzz of activity like a popular restaurant.

Doing the routine in Tucson without help, like Joe's gym at a crowded time in the so-called good old days, got me thinking about my shelved questions. What was there about Pilates that pulled me into the spa when I didn't need any more exercise? What was there about Pilates that impelled me to go to a small studio in Telluride,

Colorado, for a private session? And on a subzero day, on icy streets? I also wondered about all the changes from Joe's day to this slick studio and whether whatever attracted me back then was the same for the multitudes that were attracted now.

Were the good old days better than the modern practice? A fair question with a simple answer: No. Now and then are different, each suited to the times. Joe's gym barely supported Joe and Clara. It remained in the same space for forty years. It was not much of a business then. Had the "classical" rules of Joe's day been maintained, there would be no Pilates today. From my perspective, I think having so many people continuously exercising, so many people happily engaged teaching it, and even me writing about it are the important considerations, not whether Pilates adheres to a set of rules designed for another time. Developing instructors and creating studios could not have happened under Joe's rigid, authoritarian, unbusinesslike practices. Today many people are willing to invest their time and money to learn how to teach it and to outfit studios because they can make a living from an activity they enjoy learning about, doing, and teaching. Okay, it is a profitable business for some, a good job for others, but that doesn't explain the motivation of the customers. They are the business. Joe's "build it and they will come" strategy did not work. It took years to break through the crust of rigidity that Joe imposed to turn Pilates into something that benefits so many.

My high school friend who lives in Columbus, Indiana (population 47,000), goes to a local Pilates studio—one of two or three in his small town. His regular exercise routine has helped him greatly. Neither the studio nor his teacher, Donna, would be there were it not for the modernization and commodification of Joe's program. Forty miles away, in Indianapolis, with twenty times the people, there are approximately a dozen Pilates studios.

The studio in the Tucson spa was there with its expensive equipment and trained staff because Pilates had become a vastly popular exercise activity. Spa patrons who did it in their hometown wanted to do it on vacation. People who had heard about it wanted to try it. The spa atmosphere, modern design, and a friendly environment helped, but they do not explain why the product—the routine—is so popular. A beautiful coffee shop without good coffee won't survive. There must be something about the exercise routine. If all that one did in a studio were calisthenics or weight training, it would have a customer base, but nothing like the audience Pilates attracts.

**

What is there about these exercises, the secret ingredient, like the one in Coca-Cola, that explains their sudden popular explosion? How to answer my friend's question about why Pilates? How to define it?

There are reasons not to get hooked on Pilates. Pilates from its start has always been inconvenient, expensive, and sweaty. Although Joe's rules are gone, and these days the studios are attractive, well air-conditioned, and welcoming, the actual exercises—how one moves their body for about an hour—closely resemble what one did in Joe's gym fifty years ago. It was and still is hard work. Just like push-ups, weights, and all the other similar exercises.

Joe called his system of exercise Contrology, not Pilates. Pilates as the name of the exercise program replaced Contrology shortly after Joe's death in 1967. Joe defined his system in one sentence in his 1945 book, *Return to Life*: "Contrology is complete co-ordination of body, mind, and spirit." That description doesn't tell us much. One cannot even attach it solely to exercise even though Joe's use of "co-ordination" implies movement. It could just as easily describe playing the violin or dancing the tango or playing golf, and on and on. Even meditating requires coordination of mind, body, and spirit. Watching television doesn't.

Judge Miriam Cedarbaum did better defining the term in her October 2000 decision that Pilates was a system of exercise. Judge Cedarbaum described Pilates as "a method of conditioning incorporating specific exercises designed to strengthen the entire body, with particular emphasis on the lower back and abdominal region, while at the same time enhancing flexibility."

I can picture Joe—dead over three decades by then—in that court-room. He'd be on his feet objecting: "Your Honor, my exercises do not emphasize any part or area of the body, they deal with the body and the mind together. The mind and all parts of the body are intercon-nected and come in the same package. And, Your Honor, flexibility is but one of the benefits of my system. A healthier and happier life is the main benefit."

Judge Cedarbaum's response would have been: "Duly noted. I did the best I could with the evidence before me. Perhaps I didn't go far enough, but at least I got it as a method of exercise. Let's move on."

Despite all the time I spent with Joe in and outside the gym, and all his conversations—which were really lectures to an audience of just me—on the benefits of Contrology, he never explained to me or any-one that I knew what he meant by the "complete co-ordination of body, mind, and spirit." Or, as he also called it, the "mind/body connection." I never thought to ask. Until I started to write this book and try to understand what Joe was talking about, I didn't need an explanation. I knew Pilates had a special quality, although it was only a sense I had, like a sense of danger. Even though Joe firmly believed Contrology was earthshaking, I do not think he could explain why. Perhaps Joe wanted everyone to feel Pilates, sense its singularity, but not understand it. He loved the unexplained, the unsaid, the space between doing and thinking.

I began to ask people I did Pilates with why they liked it. My infor-mal teacher survey hadn't yielded much. I chose people who I knew were regulars. I frequently was told that they liked their teacher. I would ask if there was anything else, and the reply was the usual: "It makes me feel great." I had been down that inquiry road, and I knew that was *a* reason, but not *the* reason. Sure, a Pilates instructor with charisma might be an attraction, but for everyone? Unlikely. There isn't enough instructor charisma in the world to explain the popularity of Pilates today. And so many people do Pilates without a connection to a specific teacher that it cannot be the teacher. The explanation had to be in "the makes me feel great" response. There are so many activities that make one feel great. What exactly is there about Pilates that makes people feel great? So great, in fact, that they become addicted.

The movements leave you with a sense of physical well-being. You feel more limber, taller, and straighter, and your walk improves, all of which kicks up your self-esteem and your confidence. Your clothes fit better. You even sit and stand up with ease and authority. You and everyone else notice the improvement. Perhaps that's enough for some to keep doing it. People stick to any number of exercise routines for precisely the same reasons. But like so many exercise routines and all diets, when the novelty wears off, so, too, do enthusiasm and attendance. And when you tire of something, you begin to listen to that little devil figuratively sitting on your shoulder, whispering "Why bother?" Yet for some reason millions of people don't tire of Pilates.

My personal experience, my years co-managing a Pilates studio after Joe's death, and the feedback from the many teachers and clients I have met tell me that it is not the pleasure of movement, nor an attraction to an instructor, nor simply the benefits of exercise, nor the conviviality of a studio that draws one in. The something, that force attracting—even addicting—one to Pilates, is in the mind. The mind changes an obligation—something I needed to do, my view of calisthenics—into something I wanted to do.

Pilates, unlike calisthenics, puts you in a special mental zone. There, drudgery turns into joy. Pilates, like no other similar exercise program except for yoga, drew me in by messing with my head. I believe it is that unique combination of the mental focus and physical effort required to do a precisely choreographed exercise routine that draws millions of people in and keeps them coming back for more.

Whether you are just an ordinary person, a gym rat, or a superb athlete, Pilates is fun and provides a deep sense of well-being and pleasure while at the same time improving your appearance and your health, even your performance. It relieves you of concerns and anxieties, if only temporarily. It is like playing a musical instrument, or a sport, or so many physical activities like fly-fishing, even sex or golf. Those activities are fun. You hardly know you are exercising. Calisthenics are not fun, but Pilates is.

**

Joe's design criteria for Contrology was that it could be self-taught and then performed from that odd state of consciousness one ofttimes enters when driving. If you didn't do it at home, or at a gym, he visualized large classes with a leader calling out the names of the exercises through a megaphone. Some could do it at home. Joe believed you could eventually do a full routine as easily and automatically as walking. All you had to do was position yourself on the mat or apparatus and let yourself get lost in the task, just like Yo-Yo Ma does on the cello when he plays Bach (or, in his case, anything). Joe's method of instruction furthered self-sufficiency. Hence my solo session in the Tucson spa.

Joe demanded your full attention. He prevented distractions, including self-created ones like thinking. He forced you to turn off your analytical, orderly, note-taking, and memorizing mind. He made your body find its way to be graceful and efficient. He refused to explain why he had you do anything—or why he did anything. If you had a question, he ignored it. He couldn't be interrupted, and he remained focused 100 percent on you for as long as he thought would be helpful—sometimes just a few minutes, sometimes a full session. To Joe, Contrology was a religion. You didn't question it or seek to understand it. You just practiced it.

When you could do the routine by yourself, Joe expected you would do it at home when you awoke, something like brushing your teeth. If you did, you would be set for the day. Everything would be better, easier, more graceful, and less tiring. Joe wanted to cut you loose and wean you off dependence on an instructor. Bad for business, but that didn't matter to him. But exercising at home rather than the gym rarely occurred. Like many of Joe's ambitions for Contrology, this one exhibited his extraordinary but unrealistic faith in the power of Contrology to override a poor or insufficient night's sleep and so many other priorities, like walking the dog or changing a diaper. Okay, so folks wouldn't do it first thing in the morning: How about later in the day? Again, the conflict between Contrology and so many other demands and constraints, including the distance between home and work, made it unlikely you would do it at home. In all my years doing Contrology/Pilates, I have found very few people who did it at home by themselves. I know people who put gyms in their homes, purchased a Reformer, and used it only when an instructor came by once or twice a week. Not what Joe had in mind. Nevertheless, Joe persisted in this expectation, although he had to know from his clientele that "home schooling" was not a realistic possibility for Contrology. Even though I can do it by myself, I need an instructor from time to to time to remind me of the details and me keep me straight, centered, and focused. Even instructors need instructors.

When I lived far away from a Pilates studio, I had a Reformer in my house and conscientiously did a routine two or three times a week. I had very little other pressure on me at that time—no children to take care of, and I worked at home—yet even with hardly any other demands on my time, it was an effort to get started. My regularity lasted, with diminishing enthusiasm, for several years, but only until a studio opened nearby, with a good instructor. Thereafter, my Reformer gathered dust while I made a beeline for the studio. There is just something different about going to a gym or studio and doing it in the presence of others. It is a rare individual who does not benefit from having a professional watch him or her doing the exercises. No one does them perfectly. Corrections and suggestions are always beneficial. And getting out to a studio, like going to a movie, where you participate with others, has a special appeal.

Even though Joe spoke of Contrology as a science of body movement and added the pseudoscientific suffix "-ology" to make that connection, no science existed that supported Contrology's claimed benefits. Joe intuited the science behind his exercises. He desperately sought scientific and medical confirmation. As he claimed, he was ahead of his time, and science finally caught up to his intuition.

Long after Joe's death, when the public suddenly awakened to Pilates in the early 1990s, science crept in. Physical trainers, physical education students, and many dancers exposed to Pilates saw teaching Pilates as a career. Several of those who studied under Joe began to teach others to be instructors. Ron Fletcher was generating enthusiasm to become a teacher. Romana was teaching the art of teaching Pilates.

With the advent of sports as a large share of the entertainment market, starting in the late 1970s and early 1980s, and the substantial economy sports generated, combined with the advances in television and optics, athletes became profit centers. The care and feeding of their bodies and enhancing their performance became an industry. Many of those aspiring to be teachers had studied anatomy or kinesiology. They wanted to apply their knowledge to Pilates movements—dissect the exercises so to speak. Some aspired to be physical therapists, using Pilates as a base. Some prospective teachers merely wanted to instruct their clients with professional-seeming terms—abs, rather than your stomach or belly; glutes rather than butt; quads rather than thighs; and so on. Anatomy became a required subject for certification as an instructor. And kinesiology, the study of movement, accompanied it. Science had, at last, arrived.

***

The scientific study of body mechanics did not originate with Pilates nor was it limited to exercise. But it, too, popped into prominence as television delivered competitive sports to the masses and brought celebrity and huge incomes to the best athletes. Improving body mechanics became essential for competitors, equally if not more important than improved equipment. For example: bicycle racers were limited to the minimum of body fat—it was easier to reduce the weight on the wheels by taking it from the rider rather than the bike; swimmers had to have certain body shapes to reduce drag in the water, and so on for so many sports. Coaches had to be kinesiologists. They had to be able to examine every movement to improve speed, accuracy, endurance, and training. The need to win and the substantial rewards were compelling.

Along with the study of body mechanics to improve athletic performance, psychologists were employed to improve athletes' determination and concentration. Why did athletes choke? Why did they lose concentration or motivation? How do you handle emotional swings? Disappointment? These were just some of the questions. Winning required a trained mind equally with a trained body. The cauldron of competition was an early manifestation of the importance of the mental state.

The tennis great Arthur Ashe is credited with being the first to identify the performance benefits of a mental state described as "being in the zone." In his book *Arthur Ashe: Portrait in Motion*, he cited his own diary entry applauding Björn Borg's stellar play when he beat Ashe in two sets on February 22, 1974, in the finals of the Australian Open. "He is in what we call the zone," Ashe wrote. In the same diary entry, Ashe mentioned that he picked the expression from *The Twilight Zone*, a sci-fi TV series that ran from 1959 to 1964. Other top tennis players copied the expression (they all must have used their downtime watching *The Twilight Zone*), and from the tennis world it radiated to sportscasters and journalists, becoming part of sports talk. Today, it is used to explain the Hail Mary passes, miraculous catches, hot streaks, comebacks, the three-pointers from "downtown" at the buzzer: all those moments when you, the observer, jump up and rub your eyes to check if you were dreaming. These breathtaking moments show us what the human body can do with training, focus, and the proper mental state.

Late in the 1960s, the mental state of being in the zone and the enhanced performance that resulted became of interest to Dr. Mihály Csíkszentmihályi, a psychologist and university professor. Csíkszentmihályi's study was provoked by an experience while a prisoner of war in Italy during World War II, which mentally altered his outlook on life. As an academic, he began a scientific study to discover how and why his experience happened.

While in prison, Csíkszentmihályi took up chess. Concentrating on that game neutralized the miserable reality of prison life and made him euphoric despite conditions far from comfortable. Years later, he recalled his euphoric reaction from playing chess and studied the psychological implications, not of chess, but of the conditions that the game required. Out of this he developed a theory of a mental state he labeled "Flow." In 1990 he published a very popular and influential book, *Flow, the Psychology of Optimal Experience.* In it, Csíkszentmihályi described Flow as a mental state where "the ego falls away. Time flies. Every action, movement, and thought follows inevitably from the previous one, like playing jazz. Your whole being is involved, and you're using your skills to the utmost."

Flow doesn't just happen. Certain conditions must be present. Flow occurs "when all a person's relevant skills are needed to cope with the challenges of a situation, [when] that person's attention is completely absorbed by the activity." Flow not only enhances performance, it produces enjoyment, which Csíkszentmihályi defines as a sensation beyond pleasure. If enjoyment could be represented by a linear scale, it would appear between the two extremes of nonenjoyment: boredom at one end and anxiety at the other end. Enjoyment, according to Csíkszentmihályi, brings happiness, makes life rewarding, involves a sense of accomplishment, and is that state where the unimagined happens.

Flow is the same as "being in the zone." The terms, one psychological, the other colloquial, refer to the same condition. By whatever name it is called, that mental state is at the heart of Pilates. Csíkszentmihályi included a section on Flow and yoga in his book. (Pilates in 1990 was just coming out of its hibernation and still too obscure to catch Csíkszentmihályi's eye. But the comparison with yoga is a good one.) Csíkszentmihályi wrote: "The similarities between Yoga and Flow are extremely strong: in fact, it makes sense to think of Yoga as a very thoroughly planned Flow activity. Both try to achieve a joyous, self-forgetful involvement through concentration, which in turn is made possible by a discipline of the body."

If yoga according to Csíkszentmihályi is a "very thoroughly planned Flow activity," then so, too, is Pilates. Pilates, like yoga, is difficult and requires self-motivation and discipline yet provides psychic enjoyment. As with yoga, people are attracted to Pilates because it improves their physique, is good for their health and longevity, and is enjoyable in a deep and lasting way. It is the enjoyment that results from the concentration on the movements, the challenge of performing them, and the rewards from persistence, progress, and achievement, all of which Joe built into his program. Enjoyment of a deep psychic kind distinguishes Pilates from so many other gym-oriented activities, and it is that deep physic enjoyment that brings people back. Pilates, as stated earlier, is fun.

Oddly, there were eerie similarities between Csíkszentmihályi and Joe. Both were prisoners of a world war. Both needed to kill time and distract themselves from their confinement. As I discussed in the previous chapter, Joe occupied himself with developing an exercise program; Csíkszentmihályi took up chess. But although the activities were different, the results for each were identical: through their activities, they were able to mentally distance themselves from their environment. Perhaps they even found a way to enjoy some of their time waiting for the war to end. Prison became tolerable.

You can get in the zone doing dishes and, as Joe proved, doing calisthenics. The particular activity doesn't matter so long as it requires, among other attributes, total absorption. If necessity is the mother of invention, captivity may be the father. Both Csíkszentmihályi and Joe felt the effect on their mental outlook and attitude resulting from their activities; neither understood the underlying psychology at the time. Not only were their mental states altered, so, too, were the rest of their lives. So was mine.

**

Not once during my walks with Joe, or visits in his apartment, when most of the talk was about Contrology, did he allude to an altered psychic state. There is no mention in his book *Return to Life* of what happens in the mind. He talked continuously about the mind-body connection and wrote about "the complete coordination of mind, body, and soul," but never explained the connection, how it arose, nor why it was important. He knew that if you did his exercises with a clear and undistracted mind, you would love Contrology, and that was enough. He knew nothing about endorphins or letting go of self or altered mental states. He was not a runner, aerobic exercise aficionado, or meditator, and he didn't try LSD, peyote, or the like. What he knew he knew brilliantly: how your muscles work, how to fix sprains, twists, backaches, and similar physical ills, and how to improve your life through exercise. And how to teach his exercise regime. Joe believed that his clients loved doing his exercises like dancers love to dance, and that they accepted his theory of Contrology's health benefits without question. He knew people looked better and felt better after exercising, but the alternatives to achieve this were many. He had a personal and very private theory of why his exercises were appealing: because they emulated sex and improved sexual performance. But Joe's theory doesn't stand up as the deep motivation: Pilates is not sex, but just like most exercise, it stimulates the libido and improves performance. None of Joe's thoughts touched on the basic motivation to do a difficult, expensive, and inconvenient routine on a regular basis.

Because it engages the mind, Pilates generates an electrical impulse or a chemical in the nervous system that we register as enjoyment. These impulses and chemicals cause the brain to crave a repeat performance, and that is the stuff that creates addiction. You think you are addicted to an activity, but in fact you are addicted to the chemical by-product of that activity. You become your own drug dealer. There is no glory, no honor, no acclaim, no celebrity, nor any external award from doing a workout on the Reformer. The deepest pleasure comes from within. People do Pilates to experience Flow, to get in the zone. The addicting substances and electrical charges are generated not only by the physical act of the exercises but by the concentration, the challenge, the effort required to do them.

I understand learning Contrology and doing it under Joe's watchful eye was different from what today's Pilates enthusiast experiences. While I believe Joe's method of instruction contributed to attaining Flow, or getting in the zone, I also believe that today's Pilates puts one in Flow. That the person doing Pilates enters an altered state has to do almost entirely with the structure of the exercises and the requirements for performing them. These qualities were implanted by Joe and remain as effective today as they were when he taught Contrology. His rules, the environment, and how he taught all helped, but ultimately it was the requirements of the exercise, like the requirements of chess, that put the person doing Pilates in the zone. Joe's teaching sped or deepened the process, and his technique is worth looking at.

Joe was an instinctive teacher, what one would call a natural. I am certain that he never read a book or article on teaching techniques. Or took any course. Or even had a physical education mentor. He was self-taught. His book *Return to Life* says nothing about teaching. He never once mentioned that there was something important to learn about teaching, or that there was a preferred way to teach Contrology. For someone who expected everyone to learn and do Contrology, this is a strange omission.

There is much to learn from Joe's method of instruction. The most significant lesson that I took from him was his always positive, never negative corrections. No one ever did anything wrong, just like there is no wrong note in jazz. Joe corrected by suggesting how to do it better. Simple, direct instructions. Easy to assume that his concise, minimalist approach to instruction came from his impatience or his fixation on efficiency. He refused to explain the purpose or mechanics of an exercise. He didn't demonstrate. He would tell you what he wanted to happen, like "push the carriage out," but not how to do it, such as "extend your legs." This wasn't impatience or efficiency; Joe wanted you to figure it out, to feel and then absorb the solution. The other aspect of Joe's technique was his refusal to allow any interruption. He ignored any question that sought to find out which part of the body was being exercised, for example: "Is this for my inner thigh?" or what it did for the body, like "Will this flatten my stomach?" I once asked him, after a session, why there were ten repetitions of almost every exercise, no matter whether the movement was simple, short, long, or complex. His quick (and annoyed) answer: "Why not ten?" Then he said: "The count is always the same, so you do not have to think too much about how many." He knew that if he allowed you to take notes, try to memorize, or even stop for water, your concentration would shift away from the task and might not return. His focus on the student mirrored how he wanted the student to focus on the movements. His focus was also

Joe's way of demonstrating affection, even love. You felt cared for. You felt his concern. The feelings he left me with are still there, somewhere in my head, so many years later.

Today's Pilates, in all its various forms, still requires total concentration, still requires instructions, still requires spontaneous response, and still requires disassociating yourself from your day-to-day life and all its worries and concerns. And it provides the same physical and psychic rewards.

If the true distinction of Pilates is that it is an exercise routine that, even though difficult, provides psychic enjoyment, we can define Pilates not only by what it is, but also by what it does. Here is my definition: "Pilates is a system of coordinated movement, concentration, and breathing that fully absorbs the actor in what he or she is doing, adds grace and efficiency to daily life, relieves stress, increases circulation, augments self-esteem, becomes a habit, and most importantly is fun to do."

That definition explains why Pilates has grown during my lifetime from an exercise program with a small cadre of aficionados to one with a worldwide popularity. It is the magic of Flow, the sense of being in the zone, that distinguishes Pilates. Even Joe might like that definition once he accommodated to the modern Pilates.

Pilates today covers a variety of exercise routines. When Joe taught it and controlled it (the term was, after all, "Contrology"), it meant only what was done in Joe's gym. That was a basic routine that everyone followed precisely. Not so anymore. The movements vary; there are more exercises and additional equipment. Teaching styles and choice of exercises vary and are tailored to the teacher, the client, or the class. Every studio has a different culture and different rules. There are many names preceding the generic name Pilates. But no matter what it is called, or how it's taught, or on what equipment it's performed, it all comes from the same rootstock. The basics are the same in a Ron Fletcher Pilates Studio in Beverly Hills, a Balanced Body Pilates Studio in Telluride, a Stott Pilates Studio in Denver, a Romana Pilates Studio in Florida, and a Classic Pilates Studio in New York City. Modern equipment is functionally identical to the equipment Joe designed and hand built nearly one hundred years ago, save for newer bells and whistles and minor part upgrades. Concentration, breathing, and pace remain basic attributes. And because of the structure of the exercises designed by Joe over a century ago, everybody who attaches themselves to Pilates drops into a zone, experiences Flow at some level—always enough to want to continue with it.

The goal of every studio and every teacher is to leave the client feeling good about themselves after a pleasurable and healthy experience. When the session is over, every teacher wants to hear the client say, as he or she leaves, "Wonderful, thanks, see you day after tomorrow—same time." That's the response Joe got from me as I dragged my body from his gym after the first session.

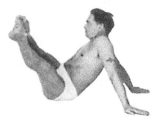

EPILOGUE

The Pilates of today is indeed a miracle. It is an exercise routine done by millions of aficionados in most of the countries of the world. Within those millions, one's color, one's creed, one's sexual orientation, one's politics or religion, one's size, one's age, even one's fitness level doesn't matter at all. Moreover, Pilates is taught by tens of thousands of people who by and large make a living at it and find enormous personal gratification in helping people.

Doing Pilates is good. It doesn't matter whether you are enjoying what you think is "Classical" Pilates, "Fletcher" Pilates, "Romana" Pilates, or "Eve's" Pilates or hundreds of other brands like Stretch Pilates, Yogalates, YouTube Pilates, or your own synthesized version. It is all good. It is all exercise. It is all something you do voluntarily and, with rare exception, happily. The possibility of injury is minimal, and better health, mobility, joie de vivre result.

Today, Pilates professionals are conducting significant research on human anatomy, trauma, postsurgical recovery, disability, and other muscular/skeletal problems. The research is being done clinically by the application of the basic principles developed by Joseph Pilates to actual patients. The results are often astounding. The research is freely shared at large gatherings of Pilates professionals held all over the world.

There are many training schools and academies preparing students for the difficult job of teaching instructors how to teach Pilates. Hundreds, even thousands, of hours are spent learning the basics of Pilates. It is an arduous, expensive, and difficult process, and it rarely stops when the student receives her or his certification. Both for the professional and the customer, the ever-present demand of Pilates to continue to learn, to stretch oneself, to reach further is by itself a life-enhancing force.

Whether you are a student or a professional, whether you are doing any one of a wide variety of Pilates with very different names, you are following the basic principles of Contrology, as Joe called it, using, more than likely, equipment matching the equipment designed by Joe. There is no "one" Pilates; there is no "classic" Pilates; there is no better or worse Pilates. Just as it was when Joe was essentially the only teacher, Pilates is not what you get, it is what you give to yourself. Joe wanted it that way.

I am frequently asked what Joe would think were he to reappear today. To answer that question, I assign myself the imaginary job of host. I would first take him to a studio where a class on the Reformer was taking place, while in another room either a private or duet session was in progress. Within minutes, he would be apoplectic. He would need physical restraints and intravenous sedation. He would, even sedated and bound, demand that his name be removed from the sign on the door, the literature, and even the T-shirts being worn by the teachers and some customers. He would try to tear down the various photos of him on the walls and, except for the Ladder Barrel (which is still exactly as he made it), would try to trash every piece of equipment in the studio. He would turn off the music and try to run the receptionist off the premises.

Then, hopefully, when the narcotic kicked in, his blood pressure dropped to 130 over 90, and he remained physically restrained, I could start to talk to him. I would tell him the story of this book. I would tell him that his dream had come true, that his life's work was not in vain. That the Pilates of today was his Pilates, embellished, polished, improved, sometimes but rarely bastardized and exploited, and that it was universal. It was endorsed by many in the medical profession, was probably one of the most frequently uttered names in the world, and was done by the president's wife, many top-tier professional athletes, ballet and modern dance companies, opera and pop singers, and movie and TV stars.

He still would not understand.

I would then say to him, "The Contrology you left behind nearly died, three times. There was no one to follow you. It survived because it was good and needed, but it took a long time to get that message out. I and several of your customers kept it going bit by bit, but it couldn't last under our management."

He would frown and ask who besides me tried to keep it going.

"My father and Julie Clayburgh."

"Good, just who I would have picked. Then what happened?"

I would continue: "We needed professional management and someone who knew your work to teach. John and Hannah were not interested. So we hired Romana Kryzanowska."

"That young ballet dancer I fixed up years ago? She liked the work, even after I got her back on her feet. How did she do?"

I would tell Joe she did great, but lasted only about ten years, and then we had to give up and close the doors. Then two more owners tried to keep it going and failed. Joe would look perplexed. I had told him what a popular success Pilates had become, but up to this point, all it had done was fail.

I'd continue: "Despite these failures, Contrology grew on its own merit. It began, very slowly, to attract practitioners who understood it and learned to teach it. As professionals studied it, worked with it, and came to appreciate it, they saw things in it that they could enhance. They, in many ways, had the same passion you did. And, to dedicate themselves to Pilates, they needed to earn a living. It had to be a business. Providing classes, private sessions, appointments, record keeping, and marketing were essential. Professional associations were formed. There is even an archive being accumulated day by day. Indeed, the Contrology of today is reputed to be the most universal and widely done exercise routine in the world—just as you predicted. And, by the way, I have had and continue to have a wonderful and healthy life because of you. Please, take all this in."

With that Joe would turn to me and say: "So now that you mention your life, and now that you are eighty-four, the same age I was when I died prematurely, what has your life been like these last fifty-two years? And what did Contrology do for you?"

"Joe, I had a very full life. Lots of pain, lots of work, lots of fun, and some success. I finally found my life partner after a lot of practice and experimentation, and we have had a great life for the last twenty-eight years. She does Contrology, even brought me back to it. I am close to all four of my children, who are all grown up, fine adults, and doing very well. We have two grandchildren. I practiced law into my eighties, was the mayor of my town in Colorado, flew my own plane, and stayed in shape."

Joe would try hard to take this in, which I understood. When he died, I was thirty-two and probably in his eyes an unformed person. He would then ask me whether Contrology helped me with my life.

I would tell him it had a great effect on my life in addition to keeping me healthy and somewhat limber.

"Like what?" he'd mumble.

"You and Contrology gave me a beacon. Somehow just putting the time aside a few days each week, focusing on my body and what it needed, and going into that deep state of concentration changed my life completely."

From the look on Joe's face it would be obvious I hadn't answered his question. He was always impatient. So I'd try again.

"I finally replaced everyone's expectations of me with my expectations. I had you in mind. You didn't care what anyone thought about you. I remembered our walks. You went at your pace, where you wanted. I pretended I was still with you, but not just going up Eighth Avenue, we were walking through life with purpose, with direction and not worrying about everyone else, not letting them slow us down or distract us, although not disturbing them. Little stuff, maybe. But for me, who was always looking to see who was looking at me, it was big. You listened to yourself and then you seemed to be able to hear everyone else. You encouraged me to listen to myself. Then I could hear others."

I would take a breath and notice something coming over Joe. I didn't know what it was, but it relaxed him.

"Anything else?"

"Yes," I'd say. "When you came into my life, I needed a model for living outside the life my parents were living. You showed me how just by your example of self-sufficiency and survival. That alone saved my life."

Joe might say, "You did good, John, after a shaky start."

I'd reply: "I hope I have done justice to you, Joe, you deserve it."

Joe would smile. If only I could take a picture of that face, I would treasure it as the only existing picture of Joe smiling.

ACKNOWLEDGMENTS

If you enjoyed this book, there are several people and one publishing firm that deserve credit. If you didn't like it, or thought you didn't get your money's worth, then there is no one to blame but me. Sorry, everyone tried their best, but I was the only one who caused your disappointment.

If you liked this book, I need to tell you it was because of the help others generously provided. My wife, Bunny Freidus, was a constant sounding board and an astute editor and critic. She shouldered my inappropriate annoyance at criticism with aplomb. I knew she was right and that made it worse. My brother, Lewis, put his two cents in every time I gave him the chance. Because he is a published author, I had to listen to him, and after I overcame my life-long competitive feelings, and I took his advice, the book improved. Paul Zakrewski, a professional book coach, dug me out of some horrendous holes. He strived mightily to suppress my inner lawyer. If you liked the visuals, if they amplified the text, then my daughter Lauren Steel, an accomplished professional photo editor, deserves all the credit. She worked hard to control my misplaced need to have irrelevant pictures (perhaps to reduce my anxiety that the text was insufficient). And lastly the team at Girl Friday Productions did what I couldn't do: turn a manuscript into a book. Girl Friday took charge of the editing, the design, the production, and the marketing, and did it with great skill and grace. All I did was write.

Turning my life with Pilates into a book on the shelf (or in the remainder pile) is only one-half the story. Pulling a book out of my head and putting it onto paper took a long time and required the encouragement, support, and periodic nagging of almost a village. I had to be pushed to go to Joe Pilates, pushed to resume Pilates after the business was sold to Aris Isotoner, pushed to write a book, and pushed to keep writing. It was always too easy for me to do something else: like my day job. Pilates for me started with my mother, Ruth. Her nudging was irresistible and like a good son, I was not an unmovable object. Thus, no Ruth, no Pilates. Then there was a gap in my involvement after the 56th St Studio was sold. Then I moved to Telluride, Colorado. Fortunately, there was a Pilates studio in Telluride, and my wife, Bunny, became addicted. So after hearing from her "You should go. You'll love it. You need it." I went. And loved it and needed it. Then came the "John, you know stuff no one else does about Pilates. And its important. You should write a book." That suggestion was timed-release. The seed was planted; I wasn't ready.

However, getting me re-involved, getting me back on the Reformer, back into the routine started the time-release. The seed Bunny planted wasn't ready to sprout, but it did germinate. No Bunny, no book, and no lots else, that's for sure.

My first audience at a Pilates Method Alliance Convention in 2007 provided the real kick start. After the talk, many in the audience came up to me and, after telling me how much they liked to hear the stories of the old days, suggested, "You should write a book." "Would you buy it?" I enquired. Some said, "Yes, sure, I guess." Some said they'd buy it if there were good reviews or if someone they trusted pushed it on them. With what I estimated to be assured sales of maybe one hundred copies, I started an outline. Then, once Bunny and my brother, Lewis, noticed I had started on a "project" (and they knew how seriously I followed my dad's dictum to never start anything I couldn't finish), all they had to do was nudge me onward. My daughters—Lauren, Eliza, and Sabrina—and son Zach and his wife, Nicole, a Pilates teacher, let me know how excited they were that I was writing this story. Mary Bowen, a distinguished Pilates teacher, Jungian psychologist, and former student of Joe's, used all her wiles to keep me on track and moving forward. Ken Endelman took time from his busy day perfecting Balanced Body's equipment to add his weight to my ofttimes sagging drive. Ken was always there to discuss Pilates history, make me feel welcome in Sacramento, and provide access to his extensive archive of Pilates material. Nora St. John, Al Harrison, and Dave Littman at Balanced Body were ever present with their friendship, hospitality, and warmhearted encouragement. My flute teacher, the talented Judy Goldwater, who as an inspiring teacher like Joe, could bring a horse to water and make him drink, helped the book in many ways. She responded to my weekly rants about the book while I was catching my breath and resting my embouchure with important suggestions and support. She found Paul Zakrewski at just the right moment. And if there is music in the writing, she helped put it there. And I happily acknowledge the sweet support I received from my many wonderful and gifted Pilates teachers: Shari Berkowitz, Amy Havens, Elizabeth Larkam, Annette Petit, and Jean-Marie Mahieu. My instructors were not only great teachers but great and devoted students of Pilates. Jean-Marie in L'Isle-sur-la-Sorgue, France, who spoke little English, was difficult to understand. It didn't matter: the cues in French, although ofttimes difficult to grasp, sound beautiful and magically convey just enough, just like a French menu.

Lauren Steel, who gathered all the photos, thanks the following individuals who took time from their work day to find and obtain the high resolution images scattered throughout this book: Kristi Cooper, Kristin Miller, Kateryna Smirnova, Melissa Tran, and Kyria Sabin Waugaman.

Ultimately the ghostlike presence of the tough, gnarly old man Joseph Pilates was the force propelling me to the typewriter early in the morning or late at night. His memory stood over me as he once had, although this time silently. He as usual let me find my own way.

As I wrote, and thought about Joe and Clara, and while I am doing Pilates, I keep in mind that it was Joe's work a hundred years ago that enhances the lives of so many. If you are among them, as a practitioner or a teacher, you know what I mean. If you are not, trust me when I tell you that in a lifetime doing Pilates, I never met anyone who didn't enjoy every Pilates session. You can't say that for golf, a vacation, a movie, a book, or a play. Or even a steak. There is even such a thing as bad sex. But "bad Pilates" is an oxymoron. And if the feelings of self-satisfaction, community, and joy experienced by so many could be packaged and distributed evenly to everyone, the world would be a better place, just like Joe insisted.

PHOTO CREDITS

ABOUT THE AUTHOR

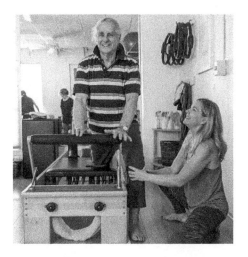

*The author with master Pilates teacher, Amy Havens,
who is making sure I am doing "Eve's Lunge" correctly at
her studio, CenterPoint Pilates in Santa Barbara.*

John Howard Steel practiced law for sixty years and Pilates for nearly as long. As one of the few people still alive who studied with and knew Joseph Pilates both in and out of his studio, Steel is in a unique position to tell this story. Steel has been interviewed in numerous publications and regularly lectures to teachers and studio owners on the history of Pilates. He lives in Santa Barbara with his wife, Bunny. This is his first book.

9 781733 430708